Rescue Your Health

How New Advances in Science Can Help You Feel Better, Boost Performance, and Live Longer

Marvin Singh, MD

Published in the United States of America by MCBW Wellness LLC

2658 Del Mar Heights Road, #520, Del Mar, CA 92014

info@rescueyourhealth.com

ISBN: 978-0-578-96892-6

Library of Congress Control Number: 2021917803

PRAISE FOR RESCUE YOUR HEALTH

"This book simplifies Dr. Singh's brilliance and expertise—it breaks down cutting-edge health information into clear, tangible steps. Since reading this book, I've become much more knowledgeable about my health and the actions needed to keep on track. I've always believed you look your best when you feel your best—I'm excited to continue using Dr. Singh's tools to maximize my overall wellbeing."

Bobbi Brown
Beauty entrepreneur, makeup artist, and Founder of Jones Road Beauty

⤫

"In *Rescue Your Health*, Dr Singh has successfully translated the evolving scientific components of precision integrative medicine into actionable understandable items. This is essential reading for all who are interested in living longer, younger, healthier, happier and cheaper!"

VADM(Ret) Richard Carmona, MD, MPH,FACS
17th Surgeon General of The United States
Distinguished Professor University of Arizona

⤫

"With this book, Marvin is giving the power to make well-informed, personalized decisions to every person that reads this. His ability to take high-level information—that some doctors don't even understand—and convey it for the everyday person to comprehend is unmatched, and he combines both education and hope into one book. Whether you're struggling with disease or you're hoping to prevent disease, this book and these methods are for you."

Dr. Will Cole
Leading Functional Medicine Expert
New York Times Bestselling Author *Intuitive Fasting*

"Amazing book that outlines how anyone and everyone can benefit from a personalized approach to their health!"

Mark Hyman, MD
New York Times Bestselling Author of *The Pegan Diet*

❧

"*Rescue Your Health* is helping us usher in a new era of medicine. While so many health experts offer the same cookie-cutter approach to well-being, Dr. Singh will help you step beyond this limited approach and to find a new level of personalized healthcare. He does an amazing job making the most complex concepts of human physiology easy to understand and empowering you with the knowledge and tools you need to find optimal health."

Pejman Katiraei, DO
Leading U.S. Integrative Pediatrician
Santa Monica, California

❧

"Read this book to optimize your health, if you suffer from chronic disease, or you are simply a curious human. Dr. Singh eloquently explains precision medicine—the philosophical approach, the scientific data and the diagnostic testing that goes beyond conventional medical approaches. He covers important topics such as mitochondrial function, leaky gut, inflammation and other cutting edge subjects in clear and concise language. I enthusiastically recommend this book to my patients."

Vivian A. Kominos, MD, FACC, ABOIM
Integrative Cardiologist, West Long Branch, NJ; Clinical Assistant Professor of Medicine,
University of Arizona, Andrew Weil Center for Integrative Medicine

"Over the last 75 years, the developed world has experienced a public health crisis in the form of a barely noticed epidemic of chronic non-communicable diseases. While the medical system has made tremendous progress in the prevention and treatment of infectious diseases, the medical industrial complex has been largely ineffective in preventing or curing the majority of our most prevalent and most costly diseases—from chronic heart disease, colon cancer, chronic liver disease and degenerative brain disorders. Here is where *Rescue Your Health* comes in. Trained in the best of Western Medicine as well as Integrative Medicine, and based on a wealth of clinical experience, Dr. Singh provides a comprehensive overview of an alternative approach to our most common diseases, based on a holistic systems view of the body and providing a personalized approach to disease. While the health care system and pharmaceutical industry is consuming billions of dollars to keep people from dying, Dr. Singh proposes a practical, cost effective way to detect early warning signs and to empower the patient to take charge of their health. A must read for everybody interested in this new way of keeping healthy and alive."

Emeran A Mayer, MD
Bestselling author of *The Mind-Gut Connection* and *The Gut-Immune Connection* and Distinguished Professor of Medicine, Physiology, and Psychiatry, David Geffen School of Medicine at UCLA

"Broadening our focus in healthcare and embracing tools and ideas that extend beyond the status quo is nothing but fully advantageous. In *Rescue Your Health*, Dr. Marvin Singh leverages over 20 years of clinical experience to produce a virtual compendium of validated advances in medical science that will clearly enhance and improve healthcare for any and all who engage the message of this empowering text. There is so much to be gained by bringing new tools to the toolbox, especially with the myriad health challenges of our modern world."

David Perlmutter, MD
Author, #1 New York Times bestseller *Grain Brain, and Brain Wash*

"Some of the most prevalent and popular questions can be answered by the practical application of personalized health in this wonderful, hands-on book by Dr. Marvin Singh. A must-have resource for the health-conscious individual trying to stay ahead of the information curve!"

Deanna Minich, PhD
Nutrition Researcher and Author of *Whole Detox*

❧

"Dr. Marvin Singh has transformed the health of many through his practice of integrative gastroenterology and shares his medical expertise to deliver an outstanding book *Rescue Your Health*!"

Gerard Mullin MD
Johns Hopkins University School of Medicine
Author of *The Gut Balance Revolution*

❧

"A brilliant and unique perspective on how we can all take ownership of our health. Dr. Singh explains how important a personalized approach is when it comes to taking care of ourselves. This should be required reading for all humans!"

Shauna Shapiro, PhD
Author of *Good Morning, I Love You: Mindfulness & Self-Compassion Practices to Rewire Your Brain*

❧

"I have long advocated for personalized nutrition and Dr. Singh has hit the nail on the head with his cutting-edge approach! The key to optimal health, fitness, and nutrition lies within our personal health blueprint and Dr. Singh does a fabulous job of helping us understand how to start decoding and navigating it."

JJ Virgin
NYT Bestselling Author of *The Virgin Diet*

"The future of the healthcare and longevity space is bright and Dr. Marvin Singh is one of a few clinicians trained to bring the best and latest medical technologies into clinical practice. Being a pioneer in personalized precision medicine, Dr. Singh eloquently illustrates his brilliant approach to health and longevity in this literary masterpiece, *Rescue Your Health*. This book is a must read for anyone wanting to take their health and performance to the next level."

Kien Vuu, MD
Founder, VuuMD Performance and Longevity
Best Selling Author *of Thrive State*
Assistant Clinical Professor, UCLA

❧

"The comprehensive and individualized approach that Dr. Singh describes in *Rescue Your Health* is exactly what we need to help heal America's broken healthcare system and can make a tremendous impact on your health today! By using precision technology to understand and optimize our body's functioning at the micro-level and taking a wider lens view of how the body's systems interact and work together as a whole, we can understand what is important for your health situation at this moment. Dr. Singh understands that we are dynamic beings, and that good health comes from the accumulation of choices that we make every day—and when we understand more completely how those choices impact our health, we are better able to make decisions and positively impact our health and wellbeing. This is the approach everyone needs to optimize their health!"

Valencia Porter, MD, MPH
Author of *Resilient Health: How to Thrive in Our Toxic World*

To Crystal, Benjamin, and Wellington for being my rocks and sticking with me and supporting me as I pioneered a new way of practicing medicine. And to my parents, Mohan and Harbans, for teaching me about the importance of helping others and working hard to accomplish great things. This book is also dedicated to all of my friends, family, and patients who helped me become the healer I always wanted to be!

TABLE OF CONTENTS

FOREWORD

An Integrative Roadmap to Better Health

Understanding the human body and our inner biology has always been the goal of doctors and scientists. Precision medicine began to come into its own at the turn of the 21st century with the completion of the Human Genome Project, but it certainly did not begin there.

It is not widely known that gut microbiome research dates back to the late 1800s and the work of a German pediatrician, Dr. Theodor Escherich. Since then, many notable scientists and physicians have elucidated the mechanisms of the human body. All of the following individuals won a Nobel Prize for their work, and have directly contributed to the development of technologies and interventions that help people become healthier and live longer.

- In 1901, Dr. Karl Landsteiner discovered the different blood types.
- In 1933, Dr. Thomas Morgan discovered that "genes are stored in chromosomes inside the nucleus of the cell."
- In 1950, Edward Kendall, Tadeus Reichstein, and Philip Hench identified the "hormones of the adrenal cortex and their structure and effects on human physiology."
- In 1962, Francis Crick, James Watson, and Maurice Wilkins discovered the molecular structure of nucleic acids and "its significance for information transfer in living material"—a major breakthrough in our understanding of DNA.

- In 2009, Elizabeth Blackburn, Carol Greider, and Jack Szostak used the foundational work of their predecessors to discover that "chromosomes are protected by telomeres and the enzyme telomerase."[1]

These advances in research helped create the field of epigenetics, which focuses on the impact on genetic expression of lifestyle factors and other external influences. The talented scientists above are just a few of many that have changed our viewpoint of how the human body works, revolutionizing science and our approach to healthcare.

I am a trained physician, long interested in human physiology. I use and teach others to use evidence-based approaches to improve health that take account of external and lifestyle factors, as well as internal ones. Over the years, I have taught integrative medicine to thousands of physicians, medical students, and allied health professionals. Evidence for the benefits of integrative modalities has increased steadily.

As we look to the future, after having experienced an international health crisis with the COVID-19 pandemic, I think we all will have a greater appreciation for (and place more importance on) concepts like optimal metabolism, gut health, mitochondrial function, brain health, and inappropriate inflammation. This book, written by one of my students, covers all of these subjects. I am pleased to introduce it.

Drawing on his expertise and experience in both integrative and conventional medicine and his study of voluminous research data, Dr. Marvin Singh has created an easy-to-use roadmap that is accessible to everyone. He writes in clear language we can all understand.

---

1   More information on these scientific advances is available at the Nobel Prize organization's website, at https://www.nobelprize.org/.

Rescue Your Health provides an overview of the wide variety of available tests and technologies that can help us understand our inner biology, recommending those that are the most cost effective and produce the most useful results.

Then, in order to demonstrate how impactful using this kind of information can be, Dr. Singh shares the life-changing experiences of patients he has treated, people who came to him with such varied concerns as optimal health and longevity, brain health, systemic inflammation, hormones, immune reactivity, cardiovascular and metabolic health, and gut microbiome health. His passion for his patients and his subject matter is evident in these pages.

As a practitioner and teacher of integrative medicine for the last thirty years, I find it refreshing to see how cutting-edge science and technology can be harnessed to guide us all toward being the healthiest versions of ourselves. I welcome this book as a significant contribution to our understanding of how we can all live better by rescuing our health.

Andrew Weil, MD
Tucson, Arizona

INTRODUCTION

THIS BOOK IS FOR YOU

When I started my own journey into health—both personally and professionally—I knew I had to look at things differently. Even though I had some of the best medical training in the world, I felt like there were gaps in my knowledge. I had questions for which there weren't obvious answers in any of the textbooks I had studied in medical school and beyond.

These questions started early in my career. I couldn't understand why I was having so much difficulty taking care of patients with chronic symptoms—which seemed to be a majority of the people I saw. At one point I even began to doubt my ability as a physician. After asking myself some very pointed questions and taking time for reflection, I realized that it wasn't my education or my experience at fault; it was the way I was *approaching* my patients' problems or complaints.

In general, doctors don't learn as much as we need to in medical school about the role of diet, mind-body connection, genomics, or the gut microbiome. This is a shame, as I have learned, because many of the unanswered questions that healthcare practitioners struggle to answer lie within these areas of study. Once I identified this gap in my understanding, I immersed myself in learning integrative and functional medicine. It felt like someone blew a breath of fresh air into my entire being. I was a new doctor—a new person, really—and I was able to help my patients become new people too!

I wrote this book to facilitate a new and different conversation around health and, more importantly, how we can leverage science and technology to get there. The research in this area is at the forefront of change in our approach to wellness, and yet it's still mostly uncharted territory. It's new, it's novel, and … it's in its infancy. But that doesn't mean that we can't start to use it to our benefit. Quite the opposite, actually.

While there may be a lot we don't know, at the same time there's so much we *do* know and can use today to improve our health and well-being. Plus, we are learning more every year. The time has come to leverage this incredible combination of science and technology to change the healthcare landscape for everyone.

That sounds great, doesn't it? But, what does that actually mean?

It means that by using the best technology available to us today, we now have the ability to make customized health plans for each individual, regardless of their socio-economic status or background. This comprehensive and individualized approach creates the most positive impact on someone's health and well-being. And we've only just begun!

By writing this book, I hope to make this information available to as many people as possible. Whether this book finds its way to a kitchen table in the middle of Iowa, or a lounge chair on the shores of the Atlantic, my goal is to share this information with everyone so that they can use it to their advantage in living a healthier life.

My hope is that this book leaves you, the reader, with a better understanding of the role that science and technology can play in maximizing our well-being, and that I can stimulate a discussion on how we can best use them to create common sense and practical applications for health-related interventions. To do so, I draw on my own experience doing just that. In these pages, I will share the best of what I have learned throughout my own career to provide you with a new roadmap for staying on top of your health—instead of under the thumb of chronic disease.

Today, advances in personalized medicine make it easier than ever before for an individual to take control of their health—to reverse chronic disease, extend their longevity, optimize their physical and mental performance, and realize a greater quality of life. I titled this book "Rescue Your Health" to encourage people to seize these opportunities. You do not need someone else to rescue your health. Instead, this book lays out an approach where *you* are your own rescuer, where you can work toward identifying what is going on inside of your body (whether you see it or not), and take action to prevent or prolong the onset of a certain disease or condition.

Perhaps the biggest problem within modern institutionalized medicine today is how it encourages the patient to take a passive role: "Take this pill and call me again in six months." If this is the patient's journey to health, it's one in which they are in the passenger's seat. With this book, I am telling you to scooch over: the driver's seat is wide open!

Currently, as I write the final chapters of the book, our world is experiencing a global pandemic. COVID-19 has touched nearly every country on the planet in one way or another. There is still so much we don't know about this viral infection and why it affects some more than others.

Personally, I have spent a lot of my time looking at the data as it comes available, and one of the things this has done is reinforce my belief that we can take control of our health, especially when we leverage the science and technology available to us today.

This virus has underscored the importance of optimizing our health, nutrition, and immunity. There are, of course, many ways we can do this, both individually and as a society. In this book, however, the focus is on you. In the following pages, you will learn how you can use the tools that are now available to rescue your own health and optimize your longevity and well-being. Of course, a healthier you ultimately means a healthier society.

Who is this book for?

It would be easy to say this book is for anyone who is battling a disease or suffering from ill-health, but that's not true. The audience is much wider than that, because good health is not solely about finding a cure or an intervention after your diagnosis. Good health is about creating a pathway to optimized health for the entirety of your lifespan, whenever you begin.

So, if you're human, this book is for you.

Every single one of us, no matter how healthy we are, can use this information to improve our well-being and our understanding of what it means to be healthy. After all, most of us will one day need answers to specific health questions, for themselves or a loved one.

Unfortunately, too many individuals are being diagnosed with preventable conditions. The simple truth is that we often don't seek help until we are already sick. Symptoms are often the final bell alerting us to something that may have been going on within our bodies for years. In those instances, sometimes the intervention is "too little, too late." But what if that didn't have to be true?

- What if you had answers before you had questions?
- What if you had interventions before you had a crisis?
- What if these interventions prevented or prolonged the incidence of disease?

I'm here to say, all this is now possible.

When science and technology combine with practical applications, poor health and disease do not have to be a foregone conclusion.

No matter what you eat, how much you exercise, or where you currently land on the spectrum of health and well-being, you can benefit from these recent advances. Learning how we can apply the best available science and technology to our discussion on health is the next step in an integrative approach to medicine and, ultimately, well-being.

Ultimately, this book is designed to help you understand the practical applications modern medicine offers from a totally new perspective, one that can be tailored to fit you, personally. Instead of using population-based statistics to evaluate your own health, you will know exactly what you can do to improve your own well-being and reclaim your health, both now and well into the future.

So, who is this book for?

In short: If you've picked it up, this book is for you, and I'm glad you're here.

PART I:

HOW PERSONALIZED MEDICINE WORKS

CHAPTER 1

Understanding the Systems of the Body

Our bodies are incredible. They are composed of numerous systems all working together in tandem to keep us alive. Even though our systems are the same, no two bodies are 100% alike. It is this individuality that allows one person to thrive, while another person in similar circumstances might only just survive.

This means, of course, that when it comes to many of the most pressing and important questions about our health, there is no single answer for everyone. Traditionally, medicine has used statistical information to diagnose and treat disease based on symptom-management of individual systems. For example, if you have a knee problem, you could see an orthopaedic surgeon who might suggest surgery. A rheumatologist might instead suggest a pill for the same complaint, and your primary care physician might go along with both. The problem is they're treating the symptom based on a single system and its population-based statistics.

What happens, then, if you're a statistical anomaly? What if your experience doesn't match the research, or the knowledge or clinical experience of your doctor? What do you do if the statistical approaches don't seem to adequately address the issue and only manage to keep your illness from progressing without any improvement?

That's where precision medicine comes in.

Before we dive into understanding how precision medicine works, we need to gain a refreshed understanding of our bodies. Specifically, we need to create a new perspective on how we're made and how it all works. Let's go back to basics.

Our Body Systems

Growing up, you probably learned some variation of the folk song *Dem Bones* by James Weldon Johnson (i.e. "the knee bone's connected to the thigh bone").[2] It was a fun way for us to begin to understand how our bodies work at a young age. While that song was only about the skeletal system, it taught our young minds that our bodies had a lot of components and they were all connected somehow, even though we couldn't actually see them.

Expanding upon that basic idea, we know that our bodies have numerous systems that are interdependent. This means they are both a system unto themselves and part of a greater system or whole. Nothing in our body exists in complete isolation, though the medical industry has a history of treating symptoms from this very perspective.

No, our body systems are brilliantly interconnected. In essence, the body is a "non-linear, multi-component, dynamic adaptive system."[3] Since it is such a complex organism, the body requires balance in order to function optimally. If any single system is compromised, it can affect the whole.

Think of the human body as a giant snow globe. Imagine it for a moment. As it sits still in your hand, it's clear and quiet. Now shake that imaginary snow globe. What do you see? You see tons of

2   Helen Brown, "The Life of a Song: 'Dem Bones,'" Financial Times, March 18, 206, https://www.ft.com/content/6d2c8b58-d1b0-11e5-831d-09f7778e7377

3   "Future Patient/Future Doctor - Larry Smarr, PhD & Michael Kurisu, DO," University of California Television, https://www.uctv.tv/shows/33132

snowflakes flurrying all over the place in many different directions; yet somehow, they also seemingly move in some sort of harmony.

This is how the body works. There are a lot of different parts all working together in harmony as one contained whole.

This means that when someone tells you that you have a vitamin deficiency and the solution is to "just take" whopping doses of that vitamin, that's not necessarily the correct answer (or beneficial). The actual question that needs to be asked is: *What is causing the vitamin deficiency?* Is it:

1. a stand-alone issue? (it almost never is), or
2. part of a bigger situation that is being overlooked?

It is uncommon to have a symptom that is so isolated that it's not related to the rest of the body in some way. Just like all the snowflakes swirling inside the snow globe, everything is connected to everything else and moves in response to everything around it. Conflict occurs when we focus solely on one aspect to the detriment of the whole.

In other words, how can we focus on the entire snow globe, while taking into account all the various components inside and how they are interacting (or not interacting) with each other?

Typically, a physician is trained to think about things in terms of specific problems within body systems. (We are even taught to write our patient visit notes this way.) By focusing on the problem within the specific system, your physician can more easily convey information to you. This is helpful because it assists us in identifying what is going on in various parts of the body in a way that is (hopefully) less overwhelming and provides a clear pathway for understanding our medical situation, or at least the appropriate next steps. This is a good thing.

However, this approach also has a less-favorable side.

Such a narrow focus can give the practitioner tunnel vision, which might prohibit them from seeing how it all comes together, or how everything relates. If we solely focus on the symptom in isolation, we are closing the door to understanding its effect on the rest of the body and its various systems. We may also be closing the door on understanding the genesis and true cause of the complaint. For example, the vitamin deficiency mentioned earlier can have many causes and many solutions, some of which would be more effective than "take more vitamin X."

Systems are the infrastructure of the body. They act both alone and in conjunction with one another. Using a systems-based approach to medicine addresses the potential gap in understanding the relationship between cause and effect.

To better understand how everything works together, let's begin by identifying the main systems that create this amazing vessel we call the body.

Traditionally, the systems we think of when we envision the body include:

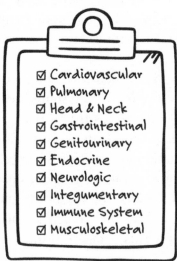

☑ Cardiovascular
☑ Pulmonary
☑ Head & Neck
☑ Gastrointestinal
☑ Genitourinary
☑ Endocrine
☑ Neurologic
☑ Integumentary
☑ Immune System
☑ Musculoskeletal

Of course, certain systems seem to have a bigger reach than others. In general, these systems impact the whole body more than the other systems. One, in particular, stands out ahead of all the rest: The gastrointestinal system.

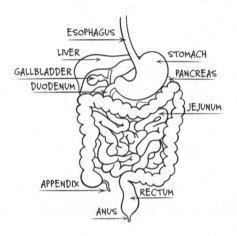

The gastrointestinal (GI) system, also known as the digestive tract, affects nearly everything else. As such, any changes we make there can have a ripple effect across the whole body. Seemingly complex, the GI tract is—to quote from the U.S. Department of Health and Human Services—essentially a "series of hollow organs joined in a long, twisting tube from the mouth to the anus. The hollow organs that make up the GI tract are the mouth, esophagus, stomach, small intestine, large intestine, and anus. The liver, pancreas, and gallbladder are the solid organs of the digestive system."[4]

Why is this system so important? Because the GI system is responsible for digestion, and digestion is what fuels our body.

We need nutrients to live. These nutrients include: water, carbohydrates, fats, proteins, vitamins, and minerals. When we eat or drink something, our digestive system breaks the nutrients

---

4   "Your Digestive System and How it Works," National Institute of Diabetes and Digestive and Kidney Diseases, U.S. Department of Health and Human Services, https://www.niddk.nih.gov/health-information/digestive-diseases/digestive-system-how-it-works

down into usable parts that are small enough for our body to absorb. For example:

- Proteins break into amino acids
- Fats break into fatty acids and glycerol
- Carbohydrates break into simple sugars[5]

These are really simple examples of how the digestive system is connected to the rest of the body. Like the other main systems, without it, we wouldn't survive.

More importantly, however, we can view the GI system as the gateway to our health. It is the single most important system we have when we want to take control of our well-being and optimize our longevity. Through it, all other systems are impacted, for both better and worse.

Understanding that our body's systems are connected is the first step to rescuing your health. We will go into greater detail on the GI tract and the gut microbiome in chapter 2, where we will begin to look at how these systems are intertwined with all the others and what we can do to maximize our health-related efforts.

While our body's primary systems are an important part of the discussion on health, there are other systems that we need to include if we want to truly understand how our bodies work. We need to talk about the systems we didn't learn about in kindergarten songs: The omics.

What are the Omics?

The omics are the *real* systems that drive our well-being. Omics are the systems that are seemingly invisible to the naked eye and yet affect nearly every aspect of our body's functionality.

---

5   Ibid.

The omics include, but are not limited to, the following:

- The Microbiome: the ecosystem of trillions of microorganisms that live within and on our bodies. These include bacteria, fungi, protozoa, and viruses. The genes in all the microbes in one person's microbiome are 200 times the number of genes in the human genome."[6]

- The Metabolome: the total number of metabolites present within an organism, cell, or tissue.

- The Proteome: the entire complement of proteins that are or can be expressed by a cell, tissue, or organism.

- The Metatranscriptome: the gene expression of microbes within a natural environment.

- The Genome: the genetic material of an organism (aka: DNA).

- The Epigenome: the record of the chemical changes to the DNA and histone proteins of an organism (aka: the "on" and "off" switches to the genes in our DNA).

- The Connectome: the mapping of all connections within an organism's neural network.

This list gives you an idea of how extensive and interconnected we are. It also highlights the fact that we have to start thinking differently if we want to take control of our health and age well.

While this is a very general list, it is certainly not exhaustive, because there are many other omics. In fact, it seems every other week we are coining another "omic" to add to the list. The bottom line is that these systems—the omics—are the ones doing the heavy lifting in our bodies. They are the systems that are really digesting our foods, expressing our genes, making our proteins, and so on.

---

6   "Fast Facts About The Human Microbiome," Center for Ecogenetics and Environmental Health, https://depts. washington.edu/ceeh/downloads/FF_Microbiome.pdf

By adding the omics to the discussion on healthcare and wellness, we begin to see that there are numerous multi-layered systems at work in our bodies. Furthermore, we know that everything works together, intertwined with one another, in relationship. As such, it's not hard to imagine how a prolonged problem in your foot can result in problems all the way up your torso—in fact, that's pretty common. Similarly, a problem with your gut can easily result in problems with your skin, hormones, and cardiovascular system, among others.

Each one of these systems—the traditional and the omics—is designed to contribute to the well-being of your entire body by working together. It's this premise that is at the core of precision medicine.

What is Precision Medicine?

Precision medicine is a systematic approach to healthcare that takes into account everything we have just discussed. It is designed to look at all of your systems individually and as part of the whole. In order to optimize our health, we must understand that everything works together. More importantly, we need to accept that a small change in one area can impact everything else, and understand that a seemingly "benign" symptom might actually be the result of a much bigger issue.

Most importantly, precision medicine acknowledges that no two people are exactly alike. So, instead of using population-based statistics to treat an individual complaint, precision medicine uses the presenting complaint as the starting point to ultimately understand the unique makeup of the individual and how their body works. For me, at this point in my career and understanding of health, I can't imagine doing it any other way.

It is virtually impossible to focus on just one system—or just one symptom—and expect great health. The body simply doesn't work that way. Precision medicine allows us to use all of the tools of science and technology to hone in on what's going on inside your body, at both the micro and macro level, and develop a protocol tailored specifically to you. It's the only approach that addresses your body's specific symptoms and systems in relation to one another.

Owing to its comprehensive yet tailored approach, precision medicine also takes into account another often-overlooked system: the Environmental System. I like to refer to this as the Envirome.

Environmental Systems (The Envirome)

Our bodies are complex indeed, but they don't exist within a bubble. Remember, nothing exists in total isolation. Therefore, when looking to optimize our health, in addition to all the systems *inside* our bodies, we also have to consider the systems *outside* our bodies that have an impact on our health. For ease of understanding, this includes both lifestyle systems and environmental systems.

Lifestyle and environmental systems include anything and everything in your environment that can affect your body and wellness. There are, of course, too many to list, and each person's situation will be unique. However, there are six key elements, either physical or emotional, that directly affect our health and well-being. They are:

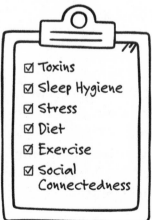

Physical Environment

Our physical environments can contain pollutants that impact our health on a daily basis. They include the chemicals and toxins that surround us, such as: mold, airborne chemicals, fertilizers, pesticides, flame retardants, and many more. As an example, some of these chemicals are considered obesogens (causing obesity), some are considered diabetogens (causing diabetes), and some are considered to be endocrine disruptors (creating imbalances in hormone systems).

Each one of these toxins could be (and has been) discussed in a separate book unto itself. In fact, there is so much research and writing about these physical environmental systems, it can sometimes feel overwhelming, especially when you are trying to address solutions unique to your situation.

So, while we won't take a deep dive into toxins themselves, we will address some of them in the second half of the book within specific case profiles. Hopefully, that will make it easier to discern what information you can apply to your individual circumstances, or at least provide you with a good place to start. For now, it's enough to know that the physical environment can have an effect on our overall health and that it interacts with our body systems. For these reasons alone, it's important to include our physical environment in this discussion.

Emotional Environment

Beyond the physical environment, we also have an emotional environment. When I work with patients, or even when I talk to friends and colleagues, I often ask about stress and social connectedness. Our emotional environment plays a huge role in our overall health, well-being, longevity, gene expression, and the functioning of our microbiomes!

In fact, Dr. Daniel Siegel, a leading psychiatrist and Executive Director of the Mindsight Institute, states that our minds are "within us and between us and others."[7] This is such a profound statement. It implies a connection that extends beyond the boundaries of physical interaction. We will look at this concept later in the book when we discuss specific case studies and the interventions I have used to help my patients reclaim their health.

I love this statement, though, for another reason: *it also describes how our body works.*

Our body is not just influenced by what is inside of it (all the organs, chemicals, hormones, neurotransmitters, etc.), but it is also impacted by everything around it. Our bodies interact with our environment, and vice versa. Within and between.

Stress, social connectedness, sleep hygiene, even diet and exercise impact our emotional environment. Just like toxins, their effect is cumulative. This means that over time, even small, seemingly benign things can add up to having a big impact. It reminds me of a quote commonly attributed to the Dalai Lama, "If you think you are too small to make a difference, try sleeping with a mosquito." A mosquito is a truly tiny insect in comparison to a human, but it has the power to really impact something significantly larger than itself by simply being present. If you've ever laid down in bed and heard the high-pitched buzzing near your ear, you know what I mean.

Just because something is small and feels insignificant—such as getting seven hours of sleep instead of eight—does not mean that it's not affecting you or your health. Over time, a seemingly simple change, such as "a little less sleep," adds up to *a lot* less sleep; which, according to Harvard Medical School's Division of Sleep Medicine

---

7   Daniel J. Siegel, MD, "The Self is Not Defined by the Boundaries of the Skin," Psychology Today, February 28, 2014, https://www.psychologytoday.com/us/blog/inspire-rewire/201402/the-self-is-not-defined-the-boundaries-our-skin

"may lead to a host of health problems including obesity, diabetes, cardiovascular disease, and even early mortality."[8]

It is clear that our emotional environment (our lifestyle), including stress, social connectedness, habits and behaviors, plays a significant role in our overall health. Just like our physical environment and its various toxins impacts our well-being, our emotional environment contributes to our overall health. If you truly want to rescue your health, you need to include your environment in the discussion.

When we understand that these external systems are interconnected in the same way our internal systems are, we can really begin to take ownership of our health and longevity in meaningful ways.

Of course, I have had patients feel disempowered when we discuss their environmental systems, because sometimes our environments are outside of our control. For example, most people don't get to have a say in how their office is run. Everything from HVAC filters to furniture selection is outside of their control. For a lot of people, this has recently—and dramatically—changed with the COVID-19 pandemic. With so many people working from home, work environments have changed significantly, and emotional stressors have taken the place of worrying about environmental toxins. Even if your environment is seemingly within your control, there may always be something unexpected that pops up.

So, now I am sure you are asking: If everything is interconnected, how can we address our environmental systems as they are related to our health, especially if there are things we can't control or unexpected surprises?

---

8   "Consequences of Insufficient Sleep," Division of Sleep Medicine, Harvard Medical School, http://healthysleep.med. harvard.edu/healthy/matters/consequences

The first thing to do is to identify 1) where you can create change, and 2) where you might need to adapt to your circumstances. You'll be surprised at how simple changes can make a lasting impact. Knowing these two categories helps significantly when creating a path to better health. For example, things you can change might include diet, exercise, and sleep; whereas things you may need to adapt to could include environmental toxins and stress. The goal is to improve things overall, if you can, so you focus on the things you *can* change.

There is no 'one-and-done' approach to addressing environmental systems. Each environmental change or adaptation needs to be tailored to the individual to be effective. For example, not everybody can afford to buy organic food or a high-quality water filtration system. The idea is to work within your means and resources to create the greatest positive impact on your health that is sustainable. Let's say that again for emphasis:

The idea is to work within your means and resources to create the greatest positive impact on your health that is sustainable.

If it's not sustainable, you won't do it, and if you won't do it, it's not a solution. It really is that simple.

When you begin to look at your environment, both the physical and emotional, you will want to create two lists. One list should include the items you can change, and the other list will include the items you may need to work with or adapt to. Here is a simple example from my work with various patients over the years:

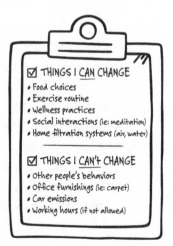

☑ THINGS I CAN CHANGE
- Food choices
- Exercise routine
- Wellness practices
- Social interactions (ie: meditation)
- Home filtration systems (air, water)

☑ THINGS I CAN'T CHANGE
- Other people's behaviors
- Office furnishings (ie: carpet)
- Car emissions
- Working hours (if not allowed)

A recent exercise with a patient resulted in the following breakdown *(names have been changed for confidentiality)*:

Sophia was feeling tired and experiencing frequent headaches. This caused her to have disrupted sleep as well as to develop gastrointestinal symptoms, which brought her to see me. Her primary care doctor had conducted a series of basic tests and everything pretty much "checked out." It was all "within normal limits," as we say.

Her doctor told her she was stressed and needed to take a vacation and break from work. I looked things over and wondered if there was anything in her environment that could be causing her symptoms. A few different types of toxin screens revealed some interesting data. To begin, her levels of mold toxins were through the roof. She also had a positive result for many other chemical toxins such as pesticides and exhaust fumes.

It turns out that Sophia lives near a busy road that backs onto a highway, and her landscapers spray her lawn regularly with pesticides. After seeing her test results, Sophia also had a mold inspector come check her house, and they found very high levels of toxic black mold in one of the rooms. Sophia made a list of the things she could change (the air in her home and the toxins in her yard) and the things she couldn't change (the busy road outside).

We immediately took steps to remediate the mold. She also installed a whole house air purifier and talked to the landscapers about not spraying her lawn with pesticides. To support her internal systems, I put her on a regimen of supplements to help with detoxification and to boost her immune system. I also made various suggestions that would assist her detox process, such as: infrared sauna, exercise, fiber, proper hydration, and several others.

Three months later, Sophia felt remarkably better and was optimistic that she would continue to improve. While her organ systems had been impacted and were showing symptoms of dysfunction, the real problem was her environment. Had she just "gone on vacation," she would have temporarily felt better, because she would have been removed from her environment. Then other providers might have said, "See, it is just stress." However, that wouldn't have solved the root cause of the problem.

After returning home from vacation, her symptoms would have eventually returned. Sophia would have been stuck in a cycle of illness, while blaming her symptoms on stress without knowing there were other factors at play in her chronic ailments—factors that she could address rather easily. Without a precision medicine approach that takes the environment into account, this would never have been looked into or figured out.

As you can see from this example, our environmental interventions don't have to be huge to have a huge impact on our health. Sometimes it's the small changes that are most meaningful. In fact, more often than not, I see people reaping the biggest benefits from the smallest of interventions. Additionally, the smaller interventions are typically more sustainable over the long-term, because they're things we can actually do, either physically or financially.

We create change within our capabilities, first and foremost. This truth has to be understood, acknowledged, and accepted to move forward.

Health is rarely black and white, as some would have you believe. There is no "one-size-fits-all" solution when it comes to optimizing your health and making better decisions. In precision medicine, health is not an "all-or-nothing" endeavor. For example, I'd prefer a patient eat non-organic lettuce than not eat any lettuce at all because they can't afford the organic variety. There's no denying that more plants—and more diversity of plants—in our diet is better for us; but you don't have to make the jump from carnivore to vegan in order to reap the benefits of eating more plants.

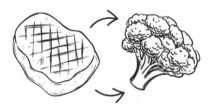

YOU DON'T HAVE TO MAKE THE JUMP FROM CARNIVORE TO VEGAN IN ORDER TO REAP THE BENEFITS OF EATING MORE PLANTS.

Good health is entirely subjective, and therefore every intervention to improve your health is always going to need to be personalized to have the greatest effect. Everyone I've ever worked with, myself included, lives somewhere on the spectrum of "good health." You are no different.

The best decision you can make for yourself today is twofold:

1. Take control of your health data, and increase your health intelligence. This means figuring out what data is missing, what data you might need, and what testing is within your financial reach to fill in the gaps; and

2. Based on the data, identify and create little modifications to your lifestyle and environment that are sustainable and, hopefully, enjoyable.

Precision medicine is based on understanding that there are numerous systems at play in our bodies as well as outside of them, and that each of these systems has a role and an impact on the whole. Knowing what information you need, in order to identify where you can have the greatest positive impact, is an important step in rescuing your health.

The advent of the integration of science and technology with medicine—Precisionomics—is what has allowed us to take this next leap forward into reclaiming our well-being. It's the best tool we have to optimize our health and stay on top of it for the long-term.

RECLAIM YOUR HEALTH WITH
PRECISIONOMICS

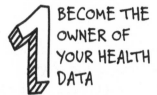

1 BECOME THE OWNER OF YOUR HEALTH DATA

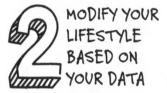

2 MODIFY YOUR LIFESTYLE BASED ON YOUR DATA

Being Open to "The New"

One of the things I have often discussed with my patients is that we need to be open. For me, this means that I need to be receptive to new ideas and sources of information, regardless of where they come from.

I recently read Dr. Shauna Shapiro's book *Good Morning, I Love You* (which is absolutely fabulous, by the way), and it reminded me of Dr. Daniel Siegel's work on connection. In the introduction for Shauna's book, Dr. Siegel describes the connectome as "the connections among the widely separated and differentiated areas of the brain." He discusses how the concept of integration has shown that it can result in the "growth of the linking networks known as the prefrontal cortex and hippocampus" and basically that "a more interconnected connectome is how you'll be achieving more integration" with mindfulness practice and principles.[9] By focusing on integration ("the linking of differentiated parts"), Dr. Siegel shows how the mind works.

---

9 Shapiro, S. L. (2020). Good Morning, I Love You: Mindfulness and self-compassion practices to rewire your brain for calm, clarity, and joy. Sounds True.

When there is no integration, there is either chaos or rigidity. However, when there is integration, harmony becomes possible. Dr. Siegel further teaches that the magic key that opens the door that leads to integration in the mind is kindness and compassion.

The same concept, I believe, applies to the human body. If we treat our bodies with kindness and compassion, and give them the things they need to get the job done, then they will do the best they can under the circumstances to keep us feeling well.

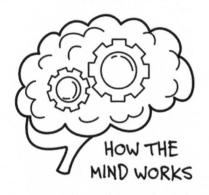

HOW THE MIND WORKS

We just spent several pages discussing the physical and environmental systems that you can actually touch, feel, or access through knowledge, science, and technology. Indeed, most of this book focuses on the use of those advances to make better and more informed choices that will lead to better health and longevity. But there is also an unseen and more intangible system that I believe is a significant part of the precision approach: the mind.

This is a more abstract concept, but it is very important. Many people may not acknowledge the role the mind plays in our overall health. Only the word "stress" comes close to acknowledging and identifying this aspect of our well-being. But I believe it matters just as much as the results you receive from any, or all, of the tests I outline in later chapters. Unfortunately, there is no "test" to truly measure a person's mind.

To better understand the role the mind plays in our overall health, I like the simplicity of this quote from Dr. Siegel: "Where attention goes, neural firing flows, and neural connection grows."[10] Basically, your focus serves to reinforce your mind. So, if you focus on something "negative" it increases the likelihood of growing negative thoughts. Similarly, if you focus on something "positive" you are more likely to increase your positive thoughts. This has proved to be true in my practice.

In working with patients, I have come to understand just how integral their mind is to their overall health. In my opinion, it should be part of every discussion we have on well-being, longevity, and what it means to be healthy. How can you truly and precisely get to the heart of someone's issues and problems and work on root cause analysis with them if you do not know, appreciate, and understand their mind, where their thoughts come from, and how they think? You can't.

More importantly, if you cannot appreciate the importance of this single aspect of an individual's health, then you have lost the opportunity to help them in the most meaningful way. It won't matter if you tell them about their genes, their microbiome, or what chemicals they have floating around in their head or their home, if you cannot help them from this mind-body perspective.

It goes back to what I said earlier: As humans, we do what's doable. We can create a perfect list of small life changes and interventions, but it won't matter if they're not implemented. In order for changes to take hold, the mind must be part of the equation.

The mind is an amazingly powerful tool when you choose to include it in the discussion. One of the most amazing things I have learned from studying the connectome is that you can reprogram old circuitry in the brain. In fact, you can actually make your connectome stronger and more capable of doing what will bring you happiness, at any age of your life.

---

10 Siegel, D. (2018). Aware: The Science and Practice of Presence–The Groundbreaking Meditation Practice. New York, NY: Penguin Publishing Group.

In short, our bodies are made up of systems. Each system matters, and each interaction and connection among the systems matters. Some players may be larger than others, but everything—both inside and out—is connected. Therefore, instead of treating the symptoms, we should be focusing on the systems. And when we think about the systems that we use in precision medicine to create good health and longevity, everything is included. Understanding the integration of these different systems leads to greater opportunities for health.

CHAPTER 2

Understanding the Gut and the Microbiomes

As a gastroenterologist, my focus has been primarily on the gut and how it can serve as the best measurement of our overall health. As I briefly explained in the previous chapter, the gastrointestinal system is one of the more impactful systems we have. Also known as the digestive tract, the GI system affects nearly everything and interacts with many different facets of our health.

The gut is the portal through which we treat many diseases.

Think of the medicines or supplements you take. Most are taken orally, which means your gastrointestinal system is involved. If your system is weak, or not functioning properly, it can't help but affect everything else. Changes made to your digestive tract impact the rest of your body.

It's through this lens that we want to start our journey toward understanding our bodies and what we can do to improve our health, quality of life, and longevity. Using the gut as the starting point, we can also develop a better understanding of the "new" systems: the microbiomes. So, let's start with gaining a clearer picture of our digestive tract.

The GI Tract

To start with, the gastrointestinal tract is lined with a mucus layer that serves as a protective barrier. Just under this mucus layer there is a single layer of epithelial cells connected to one another by a series of "drawbridges" called tight junctions. The role of the tight junctions is twofold: 1) to limit the passage of material between the cells, and 2) to block the movement of substances between the surfaces of the cell, thereby preserving their unique function.

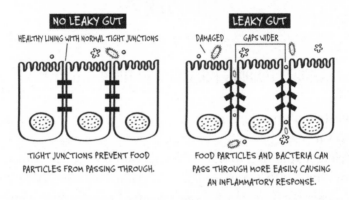

NO LEAKY GUT
HEALTHY LINING WITH NORMAL TIGHT JUNCTIONS

TIGHT JUNCTIONS PREVENT FOOD PARTICLES FROM PASSING THROUGH.

LEAKY GUT
DAMAGED   GAPS WIDER

FOOD PARTICLES AND BACTERIA CAN PASS THROUGH MORE EASILY, CAUSING AN INFLAMMATORY RESPONSE.

When there is an insult to the digestive lining caused by something like a particular food, food chemical, environmental exposure, or stress (or all of the above), we see several things happen.

- The mucosal layer thins or develops weak points;
- The tight junctions—those "drawbridges"—become damaged; and
- The gut microbiome (the ecosystem of trillions of microbes that live in the gut) becomes imbalanced or further imbalanced.

When there is a weakness in the lining of the gut, there is an opportunity for things to get into the bloodstream that should not be there (like bacteria, bacterial toxins, food particles, toxins, etc.). This is what we mean when we talk about "leaky gut" or intestinal permeability. When this happens, the immune system freaks out and starts mounting an attack against the foreign invaders. This typically results in inflammation, which can result in a whole host of chronic symptoms and issues.

So, what causes a weakness in the mucosal lining of the gut? A wide variety of things can cause the normal healthy lining of the GI tract to become more permeable. Some examples include:

SOME CAUSES OF LEAKY GUT

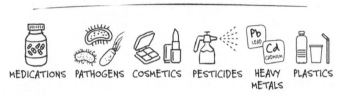

MEDICATIONS   PATHOGENS   COSMETICS   PESTICIDES   HEAVY METALS   PLASTICS

With every insult to the GI tract, the immune system gets activated and chronic inflammation can settle in any of the organ systems of the body (remember, everything is connected). Some examples include: psoriasis, heart disease, and rheumatoid arthritis. All three of these conditions are viewed as entirely different diseases, but the root cause, or source of the dysfunction, may actually be coming from the same place: The GI tract.

Your digestive tract covers a lot of ground. If we were to remove it from your body, it would be about the length of the baseline for a doubles tennis court (about 30 feet)! Furthermore, if we took the trillions of microbes that live in the gut (bacteria, fungi, viruses, etc.) and bundled them all up into a ball, they would weigh about as much as the human brain (about 3 pounds).

That's a lot of microbes!

Additionally, almost every neurotransmitter and hormone can be found in the gut, and there are more nerves in the digestive tract than there are in the spinal cord. In essence, our bodies have two mainframes: the brain and the digestive tract. We affectionately refer to the digestive tract as the "second brain" for a good reason.

The gut is directly connected to the brain via the vagus nerve, which acts like an information superhighway. Data is constantly zipping up and down, all day long, in every second of your life. The brain sends information to the gut and the gut sends information to the brain. They both work together in harmony, continuously communicating with each other via hormonal, immune, chemical, and other signals. This happens so quickly and efficiently that we have no idea it's occurring, but it is.

The digestive tract even has its own nervous system called the enteric nervous system, which many people don't appreciate or know exists.

ENTERIC
NERVOUS SYSTEM

The father of medicine, Hippocrates, rightly said that "all disease begins in the gut," and I often say that while he may not have known *exactly* what he was talking about based on today's science, he was totally spot on! He knew that everything is connected, and that the powerhouse of our health is our digestive system. Why? Because the gastrointestinal system has a lot of hardware, and all of it is connected to somewhere else in the body.

One of the most important pieces of hardware is the gut microbiome. Additionally, the enteric nervous system is part of the neural network that participates in the inner communication of our body and impacts gut motility which can, in effect, modify the composition of the gut microbiome.

Therefore, in order to have a healthy body, you have to have a healthy gut. In order to have a healthy gut, you have to have a healthy gut microbiome.

What is the gut microbiome? Let's dive a little deeper.

The Gut Microbiome

The gut microbiome is the ecosystem of microorganisms that feed, fuel, and protect our bodies. As I've already shared, the home to the gut microbiome is the gastrointestinal tract, which starts in the mouth and ends in the rectum. While a majority of the microbes are in the colon, we do have microbes throughout the entirety of the tract (3 pounds worth, if you recall).

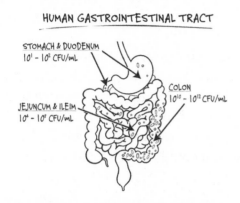

HUMAN GASTROINTESTINAL TRACT

STOMACH & DUODENUM
$10^1 - 10^2$ CFU/mL

JEJUNCUM & ILEIM
$10^4 - 10^7$ CFU/mL

COLON
$10^{10} - 10^{12}$ CFU/mL

There are trillions of microbes inside our digestive tract, and they outnumber our human cells several-fold. We have more DNA from these microbes in our body than we have human DNA. As I have described it elsewhere, "With approximately 100 trillion microorganisms inhabiting the gut, there is a substantial amount of immunological, metabolic, nutritional, genetic, and detoxification power" to be found there.[11] These microbes are a formidable force.

When you consider that a) our gut microbiome is a source for vitamins and anti-inflammatory short chain fatty acids, and b) 70-80% of our immune system is located in the gut, it goes without saying that the GI tract is an integral piece of our health puzzle and essential to our well-being. As a result, when something goes wrong in our digestive tract, it can wreak havoc across our entire system.

Unfortunately, it's often not as plain and simple as we would like when it comes to diagnosing a health problem. Because everything is connected, GI issues can show up in myriad ways, many of which can be linked to a dysfunctional intestinal lining or a weakened gut microbiome. Imbalances in the gut microbiome have been associated with a whole host of conditions, such as: allergies, Alzheimer's disease, anxiety, asthma, autism, autoimmune

---

11   Singh, M. M. (2020). Lifestyle Medicine. In G. E. Mullin, M. M. Singh, A. M. Parian, & J. Clarke (Eds.), Integrative Gastroenterology (2nd ed., pp. 599). Oxford University Press.

conditions, cancer, heart disease, depression, eczema, obesity, hormone dysfunction, and many others.[12]

It's clear that you would be missing out on a huge part of your health if an assessment of the gut microbiome was not included in your diagnostics.

This is why I ask everyone what their digestive symptoms are when they come to me for help, because the biggest microbiome—the command center, so to speak—is in the gut. The digestive tract is the tattletale of the body. When things are thrown off there, it could be a sign that something is wrong somewhere else. Or when something is wrong elsewhere, it could have its root cause in the digestive tract.

I explore the gut microbiome in much greater detail in chapter 5 where I discuss the benefits of conducting a gut microbiome test. However, the gut isn't the only system with a microbiome.

We have microbiomes throughout our body. Each one is its own system; however, in my opinion, they all work together as a whole, just like our body systems, with the gut microbiome leading the way.

So, what are the microbiomes? And, more importantly, why do they matter?

The Microbiomes

As we briefly touched on in the previous chapter, the microbiomes are the organ systems most of us never knew we had. In medical school, microbiomes were not taught alongside the basic body systems we've already discussed—and yet, it seems, they are the invisible players at the center of our health.

---

12   Ibid.

There are microbiomes in many different parts of our body. We have a skin microbiome, a vaginal microbiome, and an oral microbiome. We even know of an eye microbiome, lung microbiome, and blood microbiome! Think of all of these microbiomes as little villages surrounding the main city, which is the gut microbiome—or headquarters.

While we are still figuring out exactly how everything works together, we suspect that there must be communication and interaction between all the microbiomes, which, in turn, can modulate our health.

Personally, I like to think of these different microbiomes as different groups of soldiers at various outposts, yet all part of the same army. When something happens in one outpost, signals are released and a series of actions are taken in coordination with the soldiers in the other outposts. These signals come from headquarters—the gut—and are coordinated to stave off imbalance, which we would call illness. If one of the outposts comes under attack consistently, however, things can get thrown off balance pretty easily. Even worse, if the gut comes under attack, the entire system can be out of whack, which is why something like a skin condition can have its origins in the digestive tract.

To help us begin to understand our personal health data, we really have to look at the gastrointestinal system, and more specifically, the gut microbiome and its many functions. It's one of the key pieces to understanding how your body works and what you can do to create positive change. While there are many elements to looking at your health with a precision-based approach, it goes without saying that the gut microbiome is one of the most important.

So, what affects our gut and other microbiomes?

Everything.

Everything we come into contact with comes into contact with our microbiomes. Everything.

In one shape or another, whatever we are near affects our microbiomes. For this reason alone, it is one of the most important systems we have. And yet, because it has been predominantly absent from our understanding of health and well-being, microbiomes have been omitted from the discussion on how we heal.

Your health profile is unique, and your healthcare plan should be, too. Your gut health—indeed, your microbiome health—is a very personal thing. It's about you and your microbes, and it's about you, your environment, and your lifestyle. So, how could you possibly make an effective plan for your health and your microbiome based on what someone else is doing? You couldn't.

It's important to note that each of us are only about 10-20% similar in our microbiomes.[13] This means that as we begin to understand the microbiomes and use them as an indicator in health, we cannot generalize recommendations for the population as we have done in the past. Gone are the days of "take two pills and call me in the morning" medicine. It simply won't work anymore—not if we want to optimize our health and longevity. Medicine has finally become personal, because we now have the tools, research, and understanding to make it so.

Modern medicine is finally at a tipping point where we can personalize our interventions using scientifically-backed research and results. Over the last two decades, our understanding of how the body works, including all its various systems and organisms, has grown exponentially. By focusing on the omics, we now know

---

13 Tremlett, H. et al, "The Gut Microbiome in Human Neurological Disease: A Review," Ann Neurol. 2017 Mar; 81(3):369-382, https://pubmed.ncbi.nlm.nih.gov/28220542/

that we have the ability to not only treat disease in a customizable way, but to potentially prevent it.

I think that bears repeating:

By focusing on the omics, we now know that we have the ability to not only treat disease in a customizable way, but to potentially prevent it.

The history of medicine has never known such exciting advancement. Curiosity has always been a hallmark of medicine, so: how did we get to where we are now? It's worth taking a look back at where we were just a short time ago, to understand how monumental it is that we are able to do the things we can do today, including working with our microbiomes.

CHAPTER 3

THE EVOLUTION OF SCIENCE AND TECHNOLOGY IN INTEGRATIVE MEDICINE

Historically, in the simplest of terms, medicine evolved through trial and error. Less than 100 years ago, doctors seemed to take risks and conduct experiments based on ideas and hunches, or, more accurately, errors. Some of these "experiments" didn't work, but many did, even if it was by accident. Penicillin is a perfect example of this.

In 1928, Sir Alexander Fleming, a Scottish researcher, was working in his lab in the Inoculation Department of St. Mary's Hospital in London, when he accidentally discovered penicillin. At the time, he had been experimenting with the influenza virus. After taking a two-week vacation (and being known as a somewhat careless lab technician), he returned to find mold growing on his staphylococcus plates. Upon closer inspection, he realized that the mold was inhibiting the growth of the staphylococci.

Inadvertently, Sir Alexander Fleming had developed the first-known antibiotic: penicillin. Published reports credit Fleming as saying: *"One sometimes finds what one is not looking for. When I woke up just after dawn on September 28, 1928, I certainly didn't plan to revolutionize all medicine*

by discovering the world's first antibiotic, or bacteria killer.
But I guess that was exactly what I did."[14]

While laboratories existed, many of the gains made throughout the early history of medicine were achieved without the double-blind studies and extensive testing that we do today. For a long time, medicine was an art, more than it was a science, and it's the *practice* of medicine—the application of medical knowledge—that has done the most to help it evolve, until now.

The way we look at medicine today is vastly different. Science plays a much larger role in our day-to-day decisions, and it's only in the last three decades that technology and medicine have merged to lay the foundation for what comes next: personalized healthcare through precision medicine. Of course, precision medicine is only possible because of the advances that have been made in science and technology—and it is genomics that has made many of those advances a reality.

Officially launching in 1990, the Human Genome Project lasted 13 years before it was deemed complete in 2003. Genomics was the cornerstone that made health intelligence possible. Its significance cannot be overstated. Genomics was a revolutionary project, and—outside the recent and ongoing international collaboration in understanding COVID-19—it remains the world's largest collaborative research endeavor, to date.[15]

Four years after its completion, in 2007, the United States National Institutes of Health launched the Human Microbiome Project. The project was set up to gain a deeper understanding of the microbial flora involved in human health and disease. Phase 1 focused specifically on identifying and characterizing the microbial flora in five specific body sites (oral, nasal, vaginal, gut, and skin).

---

14 Tan, S.Y. and Tatsumura, Y. "Alexander Fleming (1881–1955): Discoverer of penicillin," Singapore Med J. 2015 Jul; 56(7): 366–367, https://www.ncbi.nlm.nih.gov/pmc/articles/PMC4520913/

15 "National Human Genome Resource Institute (NHGRI)," The NIH Almanac, https://www.nih.gov/about-nih/what-we-do/nih-almanac/national-human-genome-research-institute-nhgri

Phase 2 (completed in 2019) focused on developing a broader understanding of how this flora impacted human health and disease, specifically with regard to inflammatory bowel disease, the onset of type 2 diabetes, and pregnancy and preterm birth. Overall, the government spent nine years and $170 million dollars on this important project.[16]

The first phase of the project provided us with a ton of information. Most importantly, this information included a better understanding of the genomics of the microbes themselves and the differences in certain isolates. From this, scientists were able to develop better protocols to support reproducible sampling and creation of data. This has given us advances in how to analyze the wealth of information available, as well as how to perform statistical analysis.

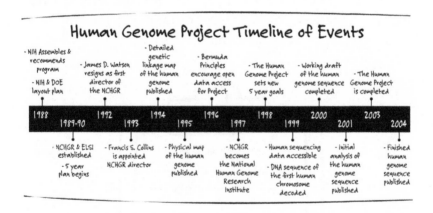

Basically, by understanding the microbiome and how to classify the various organisms, as well as how to analyze the reams of information that can be produced by the analysis, we have come closer to figuring out more and more about the microbiome and its functions. This, in turn, brings us even closer to a future where we can develop targeted therapies for specific problems.

---

16 NIH Human Microbiome Project, https://hmpdacc.org/

The work resulting from this massive project has given us the resources and tools we need to integrate science and medicine in remarkable ways. The Human Microbiome Project has set a precedent and lays the foundation upon which more research and work can be done.

These scientific and technological advances have directly impacted the opportunities we have in healthcare to make more informed decisions. The wider range of tests resulting from these two initiatives is a cornerstone of integrative medicine—indeed, of precision medicine—and it's always growing.

While the current list of available testing is vast, several stand out above the rest. In order to understand what's important in collecting our health data and expanding our health intelligence, I have listed some of the better tests to come out in recent years. Specifically, there are five tests that I recommend, for which I will provide greater detail in later chapters. They include:

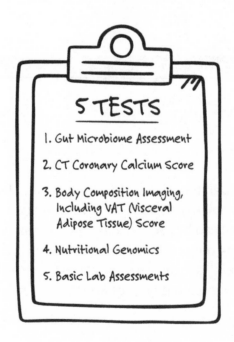

5 TESTS

1. Gut Microbiome Assessment

2. CT Coronary Calcium Score

3. Body Composition Imaging, Including VAT (Visceral Adipose Tissue) Score

4. Nutritional Genomics

5. Basic Lab Assessments

In addition to these five tests, there are others that I feel add greatly to our understanding of and access to health information. To follow, I will provide a brief and general overview of how they work, what they test, and why they're important. These tests are:

- Whole Genome (and Whole Exome) Sequencing
- Gut Metabolite Testing
- Toxin Assessment
- Pathogen Detection Testing
- Mitochondrial Health Assessment
- Epigenetic Testing
- Assessment for SIBO (small intestinal bacterial overgrowth)
- Telomere Testing
- Intestinal Permeability Assessment
- Food Sensitivity Testing
- Cancer Screening Testing

Each of these tests offers us insight into how your individual body is functioning at various levels in different systems. They provide us with information that we can use to positively impact your health, longevity, and, subsequently, quality of life. More tests will surely be developed in the future, as our collective understanding of how to test the various systems of the body evolves, but this is a good overview of what's possible now.

In the next few pages, I introduce many of these tests and provide a brief summary of what they do and why they are important and/or helpful. I think this will help put things into perspective. However, I also know that not everybody is like me and enjoys reading about all of the science-y stuff. So, if you want to skip ahead to my Top 5 Tests, you are more than welcome to do so. You can always come back and look at these later, if you're curious.

The Tests

Whole Genome and Whole Exome Sequencing

Companies like 23 and Me and Ancestry brought genomics to the household level. These kinds of genomic tests emphasize certain genes or sets of genes resulting in genetic insight or information. While they are interesting, they are definitely not the whole genomic picture, and they actually may be incorrect when trying to identify rare disease-causing variants like BRCA1 and BRCA2 (the genes for breast cancer) according to a recent study.[17]

If you want to know what is going on in your genome from a health perspective, you need to look at the entire genome. Looking at only part of the sequencing (such as your ancestry) gives you only part of the picture, which could be misleading when we are discussing health and disease. To gain the maximum understanding of your genes, whole genome sequencing (WGS) is the way to go.

Understandably, there are some important factors—or limitations— to note regarding whole genome sequencing. For example, at the time the test is run, a particular gene may be classified a certain way, but as science evolves, that classification may change. This is why it is important to keep a record of your test results and update it periodically in order to have access to the best and most current information available. A gene could change its classification from 'not pathogenic' to 'pathogenic' or 'likely pathogenic' and, as a result, the applicable information you get from a report may change with time. Many of the higher quality companies that do genomics will provide automatic updates to you, which is a bonus.

Of course, no test is entirely perfect. This is an important point to understand. For example, some particular cancer genes might not necessarily get picked up through whole genome sequencing,

---

17   Weedon, MN et al, Use of SNP chips to detect rare pathogenic variants: retrospective, population based diagnostic evaluation BMJ 2021; 372

perhaps 5% of the time or more. In these cases, when there is a high suspicion or concern based on family history or personal history, it may be worthwhile to follow up on the whole genome test with a targeted gene test for the particular cancer(s) of interest.

This example underscores the importance of making medicine personal, individualized, and precision-oriented. If I know a patient has a strong family history of breast cancer, for example, I am more likely to order a targeted cancer gene panel in addition to WGS. Also, I may order a cancer screening test that looks for cell-free nucleic acids (cfNAs) that tumors release into the bloodstream, to get an even more precise understanding of whether we should be concerned about the early presence of abnormal cells.

Whole genome sequencing can be expensive, which currently makes it prohibitive to some people. This makes the precision medicine approach even more important, because it prioritizes the testing based on your specific patient profile, including your finances and family history. But if you think about how many million dollars it took to sequence the human genome for the first time, you will appreciate how far we have come. Plus, the faster technology advances, the more affordable this kind of testing will be (currently you can sequence your genome for just under $3,000).

When we want to focus on the business end of the genome to better understand the potential of therapeutic interventions related to genetic issues you might have, then we can look at whole exome sequencing (WES) instead. Most of us understand what genes are, but how many of us have heard of the exome? Very few, actually.

What is the exome? The exome consists of the

> "pieces of an individual's DNA that provide instructions for making proteins. These pieces, called exons, are thought to make up 1-2 percent of a person's genome but contains 85% of disease-causing variants. Together, all the exons in a genome

are known as the exome, and the method of sequencing them is known as whole exome sequencing. This method allows variations in the protein-coding region of any gene to be identified, rather than in only a select few genes. Because most known mutations that cause disease occur in exons, whole exome sequencing is thought to be an efficient method to identify possible disease-causing mutations."[18]

In other words, while whole genome sequencing basically sequences *all* the coding and noncoding DNA, whole exome sequencing is a technique that focuses specifically on the protein-coding regions within the human genome. Narrowing it down helps us gain a functional understanding of what products are being made by our genes.

Finally, there is one more important point to make regarding genes. We often get excited about certain genes. But I like to stress that the body has many fail-safes. There usually aren't very many 'all-or-none' genes. One big topic related to this is methylation. Methylation is a process where methyl groups are added to DNA. When this happens, the activity of that particular segment of DNA can change or be impacted.

There are gene mutations that negatively impact methylation and mutations that positively impact methylation. Therefore, as an example, if you look at just one single gene mutation of an MTHFR (methylenetetrahydrofolate reductase) gene—a "bad guy"—you aren't necessarily getting the full picture.

It is helpful to look at other genes that might impact methylation. It is also important to check levels of inflammation and levels of certain key vitamins, along with other components, to gain a more accurate understanding of the impact on methylation. Seeing—and remembering—the big picture is key to understanding the

---

18 "What are Whole Exome Sequencing and Whole Genome Sequencing?" Medline Plus, U.S. National Library of Medicine, https://ghr.nlm.nih.gov/primer/testing/sequencing

little pieces that make it up. Whole genome and whole exome sequencing give us good information that can also tell us what else we need to look at.

Gut Metabolite Testing

In an upcoming chapter I discuss the importance of gut microbiome testing. If you want to take that understanding to the next level, you can conduct gut metabolite testing. Metabolites are the chemicals and compounds that the gut microbes create or release as the result of a variety of different kinds of functions, interactions and exposures.

In biochemistry, a metabolite is an intermediate or end product of metabolism.[19] You can think of them as the final warning that something is amiss. Based on various studies, our understanding of the relationship between the gut microbiome and the gut metabolites has shown a clear correlation between the operations of the two. As such, "one can appreciate that any substantial alteration in the gut microbiome could result in impaired metabolic functioning, immunity, and nervous system functioning, and could portend a risk for autoimmunity, metabolic-degenerative diseases, and malignancy."[20]

While investigations into the use of whole gut metabolite testing is limited, and science is still trying to figure out how best to utilize this information, the testing is available today and will only become more robust and useful in the future.

Toxin Assessment

Environmental toxicity is one of the biggest players in the game of health today. We live in a toxic world, and there are no two ways

19   Venes, Donald, ed. (2017) [1940]. Taber's Cyclopedic Medical Dictionary (23 ed.). Philadelphia: F.A. Davis. p. 1510.

20   Singh, M. M. (2020). Lifestyle Medicine. In G. E. Mullin, M. M. Singh, A. M. Parian, & J. Clarke (Eds.), Integrative Gastroenterology (2nd ed., pp. 599). Oxford University Press, p. 604.

around that fact. Today, babies can be born with over 200 toxins in their cord blood.[21] They are tiny humans who haven't even had a chance to do anything yet, and are already exposed to toxins that could impact their health. Yikes!

This isn't meant to alarm you, and these tests aren't being suggested to make you live in fear. Rather, this is another way to empower yourself. If you don't know what your high exposure areas are, then you cannot create a strategy to change them or protect yourself and optimize your health. Yes, environmental toxins can negatively impact us; and, yes, there are ways to reduce and avoid them. Like we learned in Chapter 1 with my patient Sophia, environmental toxins often remain unseen and untested until we get sick. Even then, they're not always looked into by modern medicine when addressing symptoms and causes of illness.

Understanding what toxins are and how they can impact us—as well as learning about our specific environments—can help us rescue our health. Some of the most common environmental toxins that we see today, and that I have seen in my practice, include:

- Metals like mercury, arsenic, and lead
- Mold toxins which can come from water damaged buildings or foods
- Pesticides and herbicides like Glyphosate and organophosphates
- Non-metals like acrylamide, perchlorate, BPA, and phthalates
- Airborne toxins from things like xylenes and styrene (Xylenes are found in paints, lacquers, pesticides, cleaning supplies, and exhaust fumes. Styrenes are used in manufacturing of plastics and building materials and are found in car exhaust fumes as well)

---

21 Sara Goodman, "Tests Find More Than 200 Chemicals in Newborn Umbilical Cord Blood," Scientific American, December 2, 2009, https://www.scientificamerican.com/article/newborn-babies-chemicals-exposure-bpa/

Unless you live in a bubble, it is likely that you will always be exposed to environmental toxins. (And, actually, even the bubble would probably have some toxins in it.) In addressing environmental toxic exposures, the point isn't to make the exposure zero; the point is to understand what the toxins are and how they're affecting you, then work toward reducing them or reducing their impact on you.

This is done by finding alternatives to the products or items that could be causing you toxic exposure, as well as finding solutions that decrease the environmental toxins that are outside your control, which then limits your body's exposure. By doing this you can reduce the impact that these chemicals have in tilting your microbiome toward an imbalanced state, which too often contributes to your risk of diabetes, obesity, and other ailments or diseases.

Pathogen Detection Testing

It is one thing to think that you have "parasites" or other infections, and it is another thing to actually demonstrate that you have them. Unfortunately, some providers will tell people they have "suspected" infections without conducting the appropriate testing, subsequently putting them on a series of antimicrobials that do nothing but bombard their microbiome and potentially make things even more imbalanced.

With my patients and colleagues, I am famous for saying: "If you don't know, then you don't know," and "The only way to know, is to know." While this may sound silly to say, it makes a point:

If you really want to know what issues you might have, you have to be tested in the right way to find out.

You shouldn't "guesstimate" when it comes to your health. Thankfully, there is testing available to more precisely identify any pathogen in a wide variety of bodily fluids. The symptoms are the messengers that tell us something is going on. The type of message directs us to a specific test. For pathogens, with so many tests available, it seems irresponsible to treat without testing.

This is pretty much the underlying message in precision medicine, actually. We have the technology and tests to gather a lot of information that we didn't have previously, and we need to use it. Instead of "suspecting" something to be true based on symptoms, it's better to take the time to investigate properly and confirm the data with reliable tests. Only then can we incorporate personalized interventions that make a difference in people's lives and long-term health.

Mitochondrial Health Assessment

One of the next frontiers in medicine will be to understand how our mitochondria, the little powerhouses of our cells, work. These ancient microbes that inhabit all of our cells are critical to health and illness on many different levels. Even more interesting, they have their own genome dubbed the "mitogenome" which we primarily inherit from our mothers. Pretty cool, right?

These microscopic organelles supply our cellular energy in addition to performing important functions within cellular processes such as signaling, cellular differentiation, and cell death. They maintain control of cell cycles and cell growth, as well.[22]

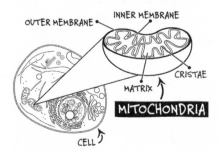

The good news here is that mitochondria are like plastic. They can be molded and strengthened through a variety of different methods. This means we can essentially

---

22 McBride HM, Neuspiel M, Wasiak S (July 2006). "Mitochondria: more than just a powerhouse". Current Biology. 16(14): R551—60.

work them out and make them stronger. Unfortunately, if you don't know how, if, or why they are weak, you won't be able to improve them as well as you could. That's where testing comes in.

The gold standard for testing mitochondrial health is by doing transmission electron microscopy on a tissue sample, like via a muscle biopsy. Since this is not the ideal test for most people due to the invasiveness, time, and cost, there are non-invasive tests that help get us close enough to assessing the health of the mitochondria with a simple mouth swab. When we can identify where the key areas of dysfunction are present, then we can identify personalized recommendations to correct those dysfunctions. Mitochondrial dysfunction has been associated with a whole host of chronic inflammatory conditions, including neurodegenerative diseases, so this is certainly an important part of anyone's evaluation.[23]

Epigenetic Testing

Looking at and sequencing the whole genome is one thing, but understanding the epigenome is another. What is the epigenome? Well, if you imagine the genome is your body's blueprint, then the epigenome is its instruction manual. It is like a sleeve that covers the entire genome just like the sleeve of your shirt covers your arm. Within this sleeve are a myriad number of chemical compounds that tell the genome what to do.

The study of the epigenome is called epigenetics. In short, epigenetics looks at the changes that affect our genes and their expression. Scientifically speaking, "Epigenetics has been defined and today is generally accepted as 'the study of changes in gene function that are mitotically and/or meiotically heritable and that do not entail a change in DNA sequence."[24] Interestingly, it seems that epigenetic changes can be inherited.

---

23 Dela Cruz CS, Kang MJ. Mitochondrial dysfunction and damage associated molecular patterns (DAMPs) in chronic inflammatory diseases. Mitochondrion. 2018;41:37-44, https://www.ncbi.nlm.nih.gov/pmc/articles/PMC5988941/

24 Dupont C, Armant DR, Brenner CA (September 2009). "Epigenetics: definition, mechanisms and clinical perspective". Seminars in Reproductive Medicine. 27 (5): 351—7.

When epigenomic compounds attach to DNA, function can be modified. This is what we mean when we say that 'the epigenome is like a light switch' and 'our genes are not our destiny.' The genome is the light bulb, but the epigenome decides whether you are able to switch the light bulb on or off.

Though I've tried to simplify it, this is a very complex topic, and at this time our understanding about everything related to the epigenome is still somewhat limited, but continually growing. The key is to understand that just because you have a certain gene does not mean that you are destined to have the condition for which it gives you a risk. There are other factors—environmental and lifestyle factors, for example—that can impact the epigenetic switches and help determine if that light bulb (gene) is turned on or off.

One of the most fascinating things that epigenetics can help us with is understanding aging and how lifestyle modifications can impact key health parameters over time. We can look at the methylation burden across the human genome and use that to help predict what your body's age may be in comparison to your actual age.[25] This is sort of like looking at the number of rings on a tree trunk and predicting how old the tree is. Methylation age measuring promises to be a much more specific technique than looking at telomere lengths (see below).

When we understand what one's genetic age is, we can track it and make certain interventions based on information gathered with the goal of decreasing age acceleration. As the science behind epigenetics evolves, this will be an exciting area to keep an eye on.

Assessment for SIBO

Small intestinal bacterial overgrowth (SIBO) is a very common condition that is likely due to a variety of reasons, such as:

---

25 Horvath S. DNA methylation age of human tissues and cell types. Genome Biol. 2013;14(10). Erratum in: Genome Biol. 2015;16:96, https://pubmed.ncbi.nlm.nih.gov/24138928/

diet, stress, toxin exposure, overuse of antibiotics, altered gastrointestinal motility, and other etiologies. This condition can be a source of chronic discomfort and can negatively impact quality of life. SIBO can also be an indicator of dysbiosis—an imbalance in your gut's microbiome—and a risk factor in the evaluation of leaky gut.

There are a few different ways that SIBO can be tested, the most common being a glucose or lactulose hydrogen breath test. This test can last several hours and is done to determine if there is excessive bacteria in the small bowel.[26] There are also other tests now available, some being blood tests, that can help us understand dysbiosis and SIBO better. The gold standard for evaluation of SIBO is an endoscopy with small bowel aspirate for culture but, as you can imagine, this is a less convenient and invasive method that is more costly. In my experience, however, these tests may not paint a full picture on their own.

In order to accurately diagnose SIBO, one must look at the patient's bigger picture, including their symptoms and any other parameters, to decide if the test results and symptoms correlate well enough to accurately diagnose SIBO. This comprehensive approach is what should prompt or suggest a treatment, and subsequently what that treatment should be. The management approach may be different if SIBO is a result of an anatomic problem, diet, stress management, GI motility, or all of the above. Using a precision medicine mindset allows us to be more accurate and effective, especially in diagnosing—and treating—SIBO.

Telomere Testing

What are telomeres? Telomeres protect our DNA's information, just like the plastic tips at the end of our shoelaces which keep

---

26 "GI Motility Testing," Cedars Sinai, https://www.cedars-sinai.org/programs/digestive-liver-diseases/clinical/gi-motility/diagnostic-services/breath-testing.html

the laces from fraying at the ends. Every time a cell copies itself, the telomere gets shortened instead of the gene itself. As a result, the DNA remains intact. Telomeres used to be considered "junk DNA," but we now know that they are more than just "junk." Just like looking at methylation across the genome, we can look at telomere length (quite simply these days) to get a gauge of our chromosomal age.

When the telomeres get too short they can no longer do their job. This then causes our cells to age and stop functioning properly, which can even cause incorrect signals to be sent from the cell. This is when we enter the "disease state," as Nobel Prize winning scientist Dr. Elizabeth Blackburn describes it.[27] Telomere testing helps us measure our age disparity by diagnosing how old our chromosomes are. Just like looking at methylation across the genome, we can look at telomere length (quite simply these days) to get a gauge of our chromosomal age.

I use this test as a volume gauge. If you are 45 and your telomere age is more like 55, we can probably assume that your body is feeling stress from a variety of factors that could be impacting your health. Alternatively, if you are 45 and your telomere age is closer to 35, then you might be able to relax a bit and understand that while your health issues and concerns are important, your body may not yet be receiving a substantial impact as a result of these things (at least not at the DNA level). While we do not yet have the ability to make someone become younger, we can work towards decreasing the trajectory of age acceleration. Using telomere length as a marker of age and longevity, we can track any changes and gauge progress in the journey of rescuing your health.

27 Blackburn, E.H. and Epel, E. (2017). The Telomere Effect: A revolutionary approach to living younger, healthier, longer. Grand Central Publishing.

Intestinal Permeability Assessment

Intestinal permeability—or leaky gut—is a risk factor for a multitude of health concerns. This is a risk factor for numerous chronic diseases, from diabetes to Alzheimer's disease, Parkinson's disease, cancer, anxiety, depression, and/or cardiovascular disease, to name a few.[28] Understanding if you have intestinal permeability, and to what degree, is important for your health. It allows you to better determine what interventions are necessary for whatever condition you are experiencing. This is a key component to addressing a "root cause" of disease. Just like the plumber needs to know how bad the leak is before he/she can understand what kinds of tools he/she needs to make the repair, this test can offer a better understanding of what kinds of interventions might be most helpful for you.

As of now, there is not a single, perfect, and definitive test for intestinal permeability, so I use a few different markers and indicators from the blood and stool to understand if there is a legitimate concern for this condition.

To try and gauge the presence or severity of leaky gut, I look at levels of zonulin (a protein that modulates the permeability of tight junctions between cells of the wall of the digestive tract), anti-lipopolysaccharide antibodies, and other proteins that make up components of the tight junctions in the gut. Some may also use the lactulose-mannitol test, which measures the different intestinal absorption ratios of the sugar molecules lactulose and mannitol, in the evaluation of leaky gut as well. Additionally, examining for patterns of dysbiosis (a medical condition caused by microbial imbalances within the body) or inflammation in the gut microbiome are other ways to root out if there could be a true concern for intestinal permeability, as can looking at the fermentation capacity of the gut microbiome (i.e.: how much potential gas production you have, based on the types of gut bugs that are present).

---

28 Singh, M. M. (2020). Lifestyle Medicine. In G. E. Mullin, M. M. Singh, A. M. Parian, & J. Clarke (Eds.), Integrative Gastroenterology (2nd ed., chapter 29). Oxford University Press.

Food Sensitivity Testing

Food sensitivity testing is a controversial test, because there is no perfect food sensitivity test—even though some may have you believe that such a test exists. If you have a true anaphylactic (IgE) mediated allergic reaction to something, testing is pretty good in this area. However, "sensitivity" or "reactivity" is not an anaphylactic (IgE) mediated allergic reaction. Instead, it is an immune response or potential sensitivity to certain foods or food components.

While the value of these tests may be limited, in my eyes they still have a place in the precision medicine roster. Even with their imperfections and limitations, it is still possible to hone in on possible sensitivities and hit a home run by making some determinations and modifications to the food someone eats by using these tests. When we do, it often helps the individual feel better, which is great—and also the goal.

When that's not the result, the worst-case scenario is that you spent some money and gave some blood for this purpose. To keep this in perspective, we are talking about making more informed food choices, not which chemotherapy you need to cure your cancer. So, all things considered, the risk is generally low for something that has the potential to have a big positive impact.

Final Thoughts on Testing

Even with everything I've listed here, as soon as this book is published there could be other tests that come out that might be great tools to use as well. This is the nature and beauty of precision medicine. It is flexible enough to evolve with the technology, and scientific enough to take into account the necessity for evolution.

The way I look at this is simple: we can wait for years and years for a "more perfect test," or we can use the science we have now to help us understand how to optimize our health based on what we have and what we know. Therefore, if there is a test that looks at certain key metabolites that could reflect the health of the microbiome, and that test could reveal a helpful piece of the puzzle, then why not get that data today? I don't know about you, but I don't want to wait 20 years to start figuring out how I can rescue my health!

Remember, one of the principles of precision medicine is not to have tunnel vision. When you use any of these tests, you cannot focus on the test alone. If you do, you'll miss the whole picture—and the premise—of rescuing your health. When you look at a snow globe, you don't stare at a single flake floating around. How could you? It would be very difficult and definitely deny you the pleasure of seeing the whole scene.

To understand your overall health, you have to use the various data points to see the big picture, by looking for patterns, building correlations, and understanding in which direction the entire system may be driving. No one test is the 'end-all and be-all' of precision medicine. It requires a wider scope and a collaborative effort to be effective.

There will always be more tests that you can do to improve your health intelligence. When undergoing a complete and comprehensive evaluation with a patient, I often order many different tests, based on their specific situation. I know this isn't always possible or practical for many. This is why I put together a list of my top five tests to help you get started, and the next several chapters will go into detail on each of these tests, as well as why I chose those five specifically.

As you can see, advances in technology have made it possible to merge the art and science of medicine. With new tests, studies, and products coming available every year, medicine is young, eager, and poised to have exponential growth. In my opinion, this personalized approach will usher in the next phase in the medical evolutionary model: Precisionomics.

CHAPTER 4

PRECISIONOMICS™ AND MY APPROACH TO TESTING

When I studied integrative medicine, I started on an unexpected journey into a world that was only just beginning to come to life. Most of what I know and use in my practice today was not taught during my years of medical school, residency, or fellowship. However, I have found that it underscores everything I have ever learned, in a foundational way.

It stands to reason that our personal makeup—when combined with our individual situations in life—would have an impact on our health. To be able to look at this connection on a microscopic level is what's new and transformative.

As I moved further into integrative medicine, I knew that I had to use this technology as much as possible to help my patients succeed in rescuing their health. What I was doing was novel, innovative, and, most importantly, effective. My patients were seeing results in ways they had not experienced previously. Merging the best of precision medicine with the omics revolution was one of the best decisions I have ever made professionally, and with it, Precisionomics™ was born.

What is Precisionomics?

Precisionomics™ is an approach to healthcare evaluations that combines precision medicine with the omics of science and technology. It is a customized and personalized approach that leverages the best and most recent advances available to optimize an individual's well-being and longevity.

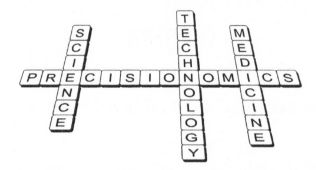

The beauty of the Precisionomics approach is in its delivery method. By using the principles of integrative medicine, this approach helps to ensure that we are always addressing root causes and using interventions that are best for the specific individual—who has specific needs, wants, desires, and aspirations. This is certainly not a "cookie cutter" approach. The Precisionomics approach is about you with solutions developed only for you.

Instead of relying on statistical information based on population data, each patient's health data is analyzed and used to develop a unique profile that informs medical decisions such as treatment plans, therapies, testing, and other interventions. The applications are vast and often lead to smaller interventions having a bigger impact.

There are many different tests used in Precisionomics evaluations; however, most tests start with mapping out the patient's molecular, cellular, and/or genomic data. It's this health data that begins to paint the picture for the physician and patient, giving them better health intelligence and allowing them to make more informed and deliberate choices about lifestyle as well as medicinal and/or therapeutic interventions.

In the previous chapter, we explored some of the tests available to us today. While it was not an exhaustive list, I hope it gives you a basic understanding of what's possible and why testing is important. As health intelligence continues to evolve, these lists will grow and change. Knowing what approach to take and where best to use your resources is key to rescuing your health now and into the future.

Of course, no test is perfect, and each has its limitations, which is why it's important to use multiple sources of data to see where there is overlap and to gain a personalized understanding of your own health. Furthermore, not everybody can afford (or needs) to do all of these tests. Nor is it always practical. "More" is not necessarily "better." Having a general idea of what tests are available will help you and your healthcare professional prioritize your approach.

For this reason, I have focused on my Top 5 Tests in the following chapters. This is a great place to start when you are beginning the process of understanding how to decode your personal health blueprint.

Each test adds value to your health intelligence in a way that you can readily apply. Individually, they offer insights into your body's overall functionality and health. Collectively, they paint a picture that is greater than the sum of its parts. Based on the current technology available, if I could choose the best approach to assessing an individual's health and well-being, as well as their risk for future potential disease, I would start with these five tests. They are:

1. Gut Microbiome Assessment (Average cost: $150-$300)
2. CT Coronary Calcium Score (Average cost: $100)
3. Body Composition Imaging, including VAT Score (Average cost: $200)
4. Nutritional Genomics (Average cost: $300)
5. Lab Assessment for inflammation, vitamins, nutrients, and hormone levels (generally covered by insurance)

These tests are relatively affordable considering the information they provide, and they are easy to do and don't necessarily all have to be done at the same time either. Collectively, they are an impactful group of tests that can quickly give you some direction regarding:

- what your risk for heart disease and cancer might be,
- what the status of your gut microbiome is,
- how your genes can influence your diet and/or exercise regimens, and
- what your true deficiencies or imbalances might be.

By starting with these five tests, we can make informed decisions about how best to support you in rescuing your own health. Collectively, they cover most of the main systems of the body, allowing us to "pull back the curtain" and take a peek inside, without being invasive.

Before this grouping of tests became available, the physician's first course of action was always a prescribed set of labs during an annual physical exam. While this gave us some information on the status of your body's systems in real time, it couldn't point to an origin—or reason—for various symptoms, nor could it show any underlying systemic issues, for the most part.

For example, high cholesterol can be the result of numerous factors that include lifestyle and genetics. Knowing your cholesterol levels is important, but being able to scan your body using the Coronary Calcium Score or Body Composition Imaging tests can tell us what the high cholesterol is *doing* to your body. In my opinion, this is what's most important. Having this information will help us figure out the best way to approach the solution, rather than just defaulting to a prescription drug for high cholesterol. Data is most valuable when it gives us enough information to make appropriate changes that have a sustainable impact and keep your best interests in mind at all times.

Of course, there's one more factor involved in appropriately using data: the physician. How I might look at the results from blood tests is not necessarily the only way of looking at things. With only lab results to go on, another physician might interpret high cholesterol quite differently. We also might prescribe different solutions—including different medications—to help regulate your numbers. Just like every other physician, my recommendations and interpretations would be based on my experience and years of practice. In my opinion, this dynamic points to yet another reason to choose additional testing: it helps to diminish the subjectivity of the provider.

Personally, I choose to practice precision medicine because of the information and solutions it can provide for my patients. This approach often helps people that have felt overlooked by today's broad and generic interventions. With each test, we use the information gained to understand your unique makeup. We then have a better chance at understanding how hard you may have to turn the dial to accomplish what you want to accomplish in a timely manner.

So, what do you want to accomplish? Where in your life do you feel you could optimize your health? Are you curious about your biological age? Do you have a family history of a specific disease and want to know your level of risk? Precisionomics can give you these answers, and so much more.

Pulling it all together and getting started

Now that we understand that the body is composed of a complex array of systems working together—and we know that there is a new way to look at health that is tailored to our unique situation through Precisionomics—it's time to address how we can use this new approach to improve your quality of life. In other words, it's time to *rescue your health.*

In each of the next five chapters, I am going to share one of my 'Top 5 Tests' so that you can learn all the ins and outs of the specific test and how it may apply to your health blueprint. Within each chapter, I will endeavor to answer the same seven questions to help you understand how you can personally use this information to greatest effect in your own life. The questions are:

1. Why did I choose this test?
2. What does it test?
3. How does the test work?
4. Why is it helpful?
5. How can the results be applied?
6. How has this test helped someone from my practice, and why?
7. What practical changes can you make as a result of having the information from this test?

By understanding how each of these tests can help us to know the inner workings of your unique body, we will lay the groundwork for an improved experience of health, greater quality of life, and increased longevity. When you choose to rescue your health, you need a place to start. This is the starting point. Let's go!

CHAPTER 5

THE GUT MICROBIOME TEST

In chapter two, I introduced you to the concept of having numerous microbiome systems in your body. However, one microbiome stands out above the rest. The gut microbiome is the leader of the pack, so to speak. It is the headquarters of the microbiome systems, both sending and receiving information from all of the others.

The importance of the gut microbiome goes without saying. The trillions of microbes that live in our gut run our metabolism, make our vitamins, and produce our neurotransmitters and many other chemicals.[29] Understanding what is going on in the gut microbiome can help us understand the status of its health, such as:

- Is there inflammation? Are inflammatory pathways ramped up?

- Are production pathways for TMA ramped up? (TMA, trimethylamine, is a risk factor for heart disease because TMA turns into TMAO, trimethylamine N-oxide, which increases your risk for heart disease)[30]

- Is butyrate production low?

29 Mills S, Stanton C, Lane JA, Smith GJ, Ross RP. Precision Nutrition and the Microbiome, Part I: Current State of the Science. Nutrients. 2019;11(4):923. Published 2019 Apr 24, https://www.ncbi.nlm.nih.gov/pmc/articles/PMC6520976/

30 Thomas S, Izard J, Walsh E, et al. The Host Microbiome Regulates and Maintains Human Health: A Primer and Perspective for Non-Microbiologists. Cancer Res. 2017;77(8):1783-1812. doi:10.1158/0008-5472.CAN-16-2929, https://www.ncbi.nlm.nih.gov/pmc/articles/PMC5392374/

- Is the microbiome diverse?
- Are there good levels of keystone species (the helpful, good microbes)?

We can get answers to all of these questions, and more, through gut microbiome testing. This information, when combined with the metrics from other tests, tells us where we need to pay attention.

Furthermore, we can also use gut microbiome testing to identify pathogens or microbes that are not good for us, or not naturally endemic to our microbiomes. Plus, we can determine how well the "good guys" are managing the "bad guys" in your gut's ecosystem. There may even be outside invaders causing us to have health problems. It all comes down to a simple question:

If we don't understand what is going on inside, how can we know— *or properly decide*—what to do about it?

Over the years, there have been many approaches to gut health that include extreme cleanses and dietary changes. However, if your decision to cleanse is based on symptoms of bloating or constipation, or if you've been told that regular cleansing is important for your gastrointestinal system, you're missing the big picture.

What if your specific flora balance is what's out of whack? And, what if a cleanse will only make it worse?

If you don't take into consideration what is happening in the gut microbiome, you're not treating the problem, you're treating the symptoms. Even if you are feeling better from one of these extreme interventions (a cleanse), you could be doing more damage than good in the long run.

Our system was designed to be balanced—to be in homeostasis. In general, extremes don't settle well. Sometimes certain practices may have a therapeutic benefit in the short term, but in the long run, we always want to be balanced, flexible, and sustainable so that our microbes don't get confused and do the wrong things.

We also want to make sure we don't create a situation where we can develop (or sustain) leaky gut or intestinal permeability. This can occur when there is damage to the lining of the digestive tract (which is only one cell layer thick, as we explained in chapter 2), and toxins, bacteria, food particles, and other substances start crossing into the bloodstream as a result of damage to the tight junctions. As a result, our immune system starts reacting and attacking these "intruders" in the blood. This, of course, results in chronic inflammation.

It is where your immune system battles the inflammation that makes a difference in terms of which medical conditions manifest. If the immune system's "battleground" is in your bones, perhaps you will develop arthritis. Or you could develop psoriasis or eczema if the battleground is the skin.[31] Here are just a few of the potential results from a dysfunctional gut microbiome:

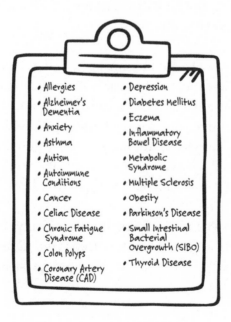

- Allergies
- Alzheimer's Dementia
- Anxiety
- Asthma
- Autism
- Autoimmune Conditions
- Cancer
- Celiac Disease
- Chronic Fatigue Syndrome
- Colon Polyps
- Coronary Artery Disease (CAD)
- Depression
- Diabetes Mellitus
- Eczema
- Inflammatory Bowel Disease
- Metabolic Syndrome
- Multiple Sclerosis
- Obesity
- Parkinson's Disease
- Small Intestinal Bacterial Overgrowth (SIBO)
- Thyroid Disease

---

31   Singh, M. M. (2017). Diet, Environmental Chemicals, and the Gut Microbiome. In A. Cohen & F. S. Vom Saal (Eds.), Integrative Environmental Medicine (1st ed., ch 6). Oxford University Press.

Dysbiosis, or an imbalance in the gut microbiome, is associated with many different conditions and health problems, such as the ones listed above. It is very important to understand how to optimize gut health so that we can address these imbalances and risks for a variety of conditions, many of which may not even develop for years.

Regardless of where these diseases and conditions manifest, hopefully you have grasped that different diseases and conditions can all originate in the same place: the gut. As such, we can now appreciate how "any substantial alteration in the gut microbiome could result in impaired metabolic functioning, immunity, and nervous system functioning, and could portend a risk for autoimmunity, metabolic-degenerative diseases, and malignancy as a result of the derangements that occur."[32]

At this point in time, we have tests that will list out some or all of the microbes in our gut, which is great! However, sequencing the gut microbiome is not enough on its own. Understanding how to interpret the information is key.

You can't just look at some blood work and a list of your genes and get a complete picture, nor can you "standardize" the results based on population statistics, because our gut microbiomes are only 10-20% similar. The overlap between individuals is tiny. In a recent study, "almost 10 million microbial genes were recently identified in 1,267 fecal samples, of which about only 300,000 are shared between more than 50% of the individuals."[33]

Outside of identifying a direct pathogen (a really "bad guy") that is thought to be the reason for symptoms you might have, simply having a list of what is in the gut microbiome isn't enough. This

---

32 Singh, M. M. (2020). Lifestyle Medicine. In G. E. Mullin, M. M. Singh, A. M. Parian, & J. Clarke (Eds.), Integrative Gastroenterology (2nd ed., pp. 599). Oxford University Press, p. 604.

33 Zhu, A., Sunagawa, S., Mende, D.R. et al. Inter-individual differences in the gene content of human gut bacterial species. Genome Biol 16, 82 (2015). https://doi.org/10.1186/s13059-015-0646-9; see also Gilbert JA. Our unique microbial identity. Genome Biol. 2015;16(1):97. Published 2015 May 14, https://www.ncbi.nlm.nih.gov/pmc/articles/PMC4430908/

means that while we want to know who is at the party, what we really need to know is how good the party is. We want to know:

- how diverse the ecosystem is,
- how resilient it is,
- how well it can keep balance,
- how much inflammation is going on, and
- what sort of products are (or are not) being produced by the collective system.

When you focus solely on the list of microbes in the system, you lose the opportunity to really understand what's going on. For example, you could have one "bad guy" in the microbiome, but 100 "good guys." If the "good guys" are controlling and suppressing the "bad guy" well enough that it isn't doing any harm to the system, the system maintains balance. In this scenario, there would be no point in focusing entirely on the "bad guy" simply because it made the list, nor would it be particularly helpful to choose an intervention based solely on its presence.

Of course, if there are pathogens, it is important to address any dysfunction in the microbiome directly. By knowing the *composition* of the gut microbiome, we can do this more effectively, which also makes potential interventions more successful and sustainable.

In general, we need to stop thinking of health as a "program" or "diet," and instead focus on what is necessary to make a paradigm shift. Programs and diets have a set start and end point, health does not. Furthermore, the microbiome does not either.

The microbiome persists always, all day, every day. Shifts and changes occur all the time. Remember, everything that comes into contact with our microbiome impacts it. Everything. The system is designed to be ever-changing and adaptable. While a diet or program may create some temporary changes, it is important to understand their impact on the system as a whole (whether it's positive or negative), and what can be done to continually optimize it. As the human hosts, we need to be flexible enough to understand the microbiome and then act on that understanding on a regular basis.

The Gut Microbiome test empowers us to do just that.

Why did I choose this test?

Given the advances in technology which have allowed us to reduce the cost of a comprehensive microbiome analysis, this test is now affordable, widely available, and easy to do. You will want to make sure the company you are using to do the test is offering *whole microbiome genome sequencing,* not just giving you a list of a handful of microbes.

It wouldn't make sense to make decisions for the entire population of the planet by only focusing on one neighborhood in one city. No, you need a good picture of the *entire* ecosystem. A whole gut microbiome test gives you that, is easily done, and is the best way of understanding what is going on inside of your body specifically.

What does it test?

The test looks for genetic material in your stool from all the various microbes and then sequences their genetic material for the purpose of identifying the organisms. Additionally, the Gut Microbiome test is among the tests that offer insight into what processes are going on in the microbiome. This means that, among many other factors, we can understand

- the degree of inflammation,
- how food is being digested,

- what might be missing,
- what might be in excess,
- how diverse the microbiome is, and
- how strong the microbiome is.

This test is the best way to get a comprehensive and personal look at your gut health and the specific functioning of your gut microbiome.

How does the test work?

Generally, you will take a stool sample and submit it to the lab for analysis. There is some continuing concern over the accuracy of testing the entire microbiome, because the samples may be more reflective of the rectal microbiome as opposed to the microbiome of the entire gut. While this concern is understandable, the test methodologies are continually evolving, and important information can still be gleaned. The better tests may be those that request sampling from multiple sites of the stool sample and even a core sample from the stool.

Why is the test helpful?

This test paints a much broader picture than anything we can get any other way. By using the Gut Microbiome test, we can identify what microbes are present and what their activity is. This can help us understand the overall health and stability of your gut microbiome, which is a key player in understanding your overall health. It's one of the best places to start if you are experiencing symptoms elsewhere, as we have already mentioned, because imbalance in the gut microbiome can create imbalance elsewhere.

How can the test results be applied?

Your results can be used to suggest certain treatments or supplements that can heal your gut lining and improve the health of your microbiome. Together, we can create personalized nutrition plans and lifestyle plans that are aimed at positively impacting your personal microbiome, not someone else's. By retesting and rechecking, we can see actual results from the changes that have been made, including what improvements have been made and where further adjustments may be necessary.

The gut microbiome is always going to be shifting and changing, no matter what, whether we want it to or not. Accepting this simple truth can only help you in rescuing your health. By staying on top of your gut health, evaluating it, and adjusting your lifestyle and other factors as a result, you will be one step ahead. Having the knowledge to positively influence your risk profile will help you to have a better quality of life and a longer length of life, ideally as a healthier individual.

How has this test helped someone from my practice, and why?

A few years ago, I worked with a patient who had multiple autoimmune diseases and several gastrointestinal symptoms. Part of her initial evaluation involved looking into her gut microbiome. After we identified some key imbalances in her system, the first step was to help her modify her diet based on our findings, as well as to support her with gut healing supplements and herbs. After this first phase of changes, we addressed ways to improve her sleep hygiene, reduce her toxin exposure, and optimize how she manages stress.

About three months later, she called me with much excitement in her voice, saying she could not wait until her follow up visit to tell me how good she was feeling. It had taken a few months before she started noticing substantial changes, but with persistence and patience her efforts paid off. She noticed that her joints were no longer stiff in the morning, her fibromyalgia pains didn't bother her anymore, and she had no more bloating or constipation.

These improvements to her quality of life empowered her in such a way that it prompted her to learn about meditation, take a cooking class, and help others with symptoms similar to hers.

This is a great example of how health can snowball into control (through empowerment), just as easily as it can snowball out of control (through frustration). This is why Precisionomics works; it is the pathway to rescuing *your* health.

What practical changes can you make as a result of having the information from this test?

Data from the gut microbiome test can be used in a variety of ways, each of which can have a positive impact on your quality of life. Some of the interventions and positive impacts include:

- diet and lifestyle changes
- supplements and medication management
- symptoms management
- weight loss
- improved mental acuity
- reduced inflammation
- reduction in risk for chronic disease
- management of symptoms related to chronic inflammation and chronic disease

Understanding the health and functionality of the gut microbiome is one of the key steps to understanding your overall health, since it informs and impacts so much of the rest of your body. This is why the Gut Microbiome test is one of my Top 5 Tests and my go-to when assessing a new patient.

CHAPTER 6

THE HEART SCAN

The second of my top five recommended tests is the CT Coronary Calcium Scan. What is a CT Coronary Calcium Scan? Well, the Mayo Clinic defines it as:

> *A specialized X-ray test that provides pictures of your heart that can help your doctor detect and measure calcium-containing plaque in the arteries.*[34]

An easier way to explain it is to say that we're looking at the "plumbing" related to your heart to see if there are any "clogs" or build-up. Just as the plumbing in our homes can get clogged from years of grease and debris, our heart's plumbing can have a build-up as well. This build-up becomes plaque on the artery walls, which slows the flow of blood to the rest of the body while also increasing the pressure (hence, we get high blood pressure, or hypertension).

Think of a hose. If the hose narrows, less water is able to go through. So, if you're pumping the same volume of water at the same rate, it has to be pushed through at a higher pressure, kind of like a pressure washer. It's great for cleaning out your gutters or scouring your patio, but it's not great for your cardiovascular system.

---

34 Heart Scan (Coronary Calcium Scan), Mayo Clinic, https://www.mayoclinic.org/tests-procedures/heart-scan/about/pac-20384686

How do we develop plaque? Again, the Mayo Clinic has a great explanation:

> *Plaque is made up of fats, cholesterol, calcium and other substances in the blood. It develops gradually over time, long before there are any signs or symptoms of disease. These deposits can restrict the flow of oxygen-rich blood to the muscles of the heart. Plaque also may burst, triggering a blood clot that can cause a heart attack.*[35]

Clearly, you don't want a lot of plaque building up in your arteries.

This test, which is essentially a quick, low radiation CT scan, can be done in conjunction with other non-invasive cardiac imaging (like a cardiac MRI or echocardiogram) to detect structural problems in the heart and understand what your risk is for cardiovascular disease that you might not know you had. This test allows us to see how the heart is working and what the plaque burden may be so that we don't wait until after we have a problem to investigate.

Some people express concerns at the radiation exposure necessary to conduct this test, especially since it is elective. However, the low level of radiation (similar to an X-ray) is 100% worth the information you will gather, especially if it alerts you to a problem before it becomes a fatal one.

Unfortunately, there are plenty of people who have moderate-to-severe coronary artery disease risk and don't know it, at least not until they collapse unexpectedly from a heart attack. Too often, people who look physically healthy are anything but. This would be your classic case of a thin person, one who exercises and appears to be well on the outside, suddenly having a major heart attack "out of the blue."

---

35 Ibid.

Unfortunately, it's rarely out of the blue, and regular imaging can prevent a lot of these traumatic events from happening. Knowing the functionality of your heart—including your coronary calcium score—allows us to intervene before lack of functionality becomes a problem, and usually with a much simpler solution.

This test will provide you with a CT coronary calcium score. In general, a score of 0 is very low risk; 1-99 is mildly increased risk; 100-299 is moderately increased risk; and 300 or greater is moderate-to-severely increased risk.[36]

The following chart clearly outlines the various categories:

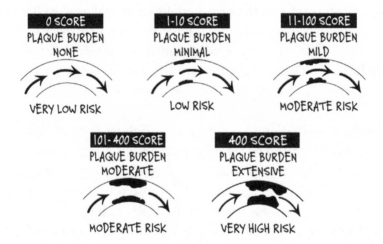

One of the hallmarks of Precisionomics is the desire to know what is going on before something happens. We want to know if you *could* have a heart attack, before you have a heart attack. It seems counterintuitive to wait until you have chest pain or your first heart attack to start optimizing your health. The damage to your heart will already have been done.

36 Divakaran S, Cheezum MK, Hulten EA, et al. Use of cardiac CT and calcium scoring for detecting coronary plaque: implications on prognosis and patient management. Br J Radiol. 2015;88(1046), https://www.ncbi.nlm.nih.gov/pmc/articles/PMC4614250/

Furthermore, you may end up needing medications or developing other problems as a result of your first heart attack. Since we also know that much of this risk starts when we are younger—before the concept of a heart attack even enters our minds—a test like the CT Coronary Calcium Scan can really be a game-changer in rescuing your health.

Why did I choose this test?

The CT Coronary Calcium Scan is a great way to determine what your cardiac risk is. It is an inexpensive—and non-invasive—way of knowing what is going on inside your coronary arteries so that we can better understand what your risk of heart disease and heart attack may be. The risk-benefit ratio makes it well worth doing this test, especially if you have any family history of heart disease, pre-diabetes, metabolic syndrome, insulin resistance, or even have developed diabetes. Knowing your coronary health is an important piece of your wellness puzzle.

To underscore that point, a recent study published by the National Institutes of Health (NIH) suggested a high prevalence of heart disease in young, asymptomatic people with diabetes, as diagnosed by the CT Coronary Calcium test.[37] These results emphasize the point that heart disease really can be a silent killer and that most symptoms go undetected for years before there is a noticeable problem. Intervening earlier is now possible with the CT Coronary Calcium Scan.

What does it test?

Essentially, the test assesses the blood flow in and out of the heart by looking at the coronary arteries. This specialized CT Scan measures calcium-containing plaque or build-up in your coronary arteries by taking a picture of your heart and its surrounding

---

37 Siddiqi Z et al, Coronary Artery Calcium Score as a Predictor of Cardiovascular Risk in Asymptomatic Patients of Type 2 Diabetes. J Assoc Physicians India. 2020 Feb;68(2):23-26, https://www.ncbi.nlm.nih.gov/pubmed/32009357

blood vessels. I've already mentioned how, when plaque builds up, it slows down blood flow by narrowing the artery. Of course, when blood doesn't flow well, the heart and the body don't get as much blood as they need.

Without proper intervention, as the blood flow continues to decrease, you can develop shortness of breath, chest pain, heart dysfunction, and eventually, a heart attack. This test will give you and your doctor quantifiable data that you can use to properly address this hidden cause of disease.

How does the test work?

The Coronary Calcium Scan is a "CAT scan" (or CT- Computerized Tomography) that is non-invasive, requiring no contrast or IV. It is a specialized type of X-ray that takes about 30 minutes to conduct. Similar to an X-ray, it 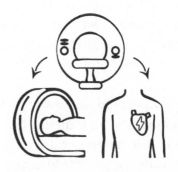 lets us see what's going on inside your body, by creating multislice and multiple cross-section images of the plaque deposits in your blood vessels.

Why is it helpful?

This test is one of the easiest, least expensive (average cost of $100 or less), and fastest non-invasive ways to gain an understanding of your risk for heart disease. It can give you and your doctor a clearer understanding of your health, even if you are asymptomatic and feel fine. Most importantly, however, it can help you make smaller, more impactful and effective interventions earlier on, potentially staving off the need for a major surgery—or major life changes—later.

How can the results be applied?

Based on your calcium score, your doctor will help formulate a plan that can reduce your risk for having a heart attack. In some cases, this may include medications, and it should always include integrative and lifestyle measures to improve your health and *reverse* your risk.

Yes, this is reversible!

As long ago as 1998, Dr. Dean Ornish published an article in the Journal of the American Medical Association outlining how regression of coronary atherosclerosis (build-up of plaque in the arteries) was possible with intensive lifestyle changes.[38] Mainstream medicine has taken a little longer to come around to this concept, but it seems everyone is now firmly on board.

The key point to take away from this article is that it if you give your body the ingredients that it needs and wants, it will do the best that it can under its circumstances. Your body wants to be well. Your body wants to heal, and your body wants you to *rescue your health.*

If you gather the data, such as your CT Coronary Calcium Score, and create appropriate interventions early on, your body will reward you in return. The main problem we face in rescuing our health is not knowing how to rescue it. We have no way of truly knowing if we are doing the right things or if our prior habits and experiences have already contributed to—or created—a problem. That's why a test like this should be done. It's easy and can give us insight into answering these questions. It can also provide a roadmap to better health as well as validation that the changes we are making are working.

---

38 Ornish, D, et al, Intensive Lifestyle Changes for Reversal of Coronary Heart Disease, JAMA, December 16, 1998—Vol 280, No. 23, 2000-2007, https://www.ornish.com/wp-content/uploads/Intensive-lifestyle-changes-for-reversal-of-coronary-heart-disease1.pdf

How has this test helped someone from my practice, and why?

Several years ago, I worked with a middle-aged male patient who thought he was "healthy." He was a busy professional who did the best he could as much of the time as possible. Maybe he indulged a little bit every once in a while, "But who doesn't?" he said.

As part of his evaluation, we conducted a CT Coronary Calcium Scan, and his result was 110. According to the Mayo Clinic, the score "reflects the total area of calcium deposits and the density of the calcium," as follows:[39]

- A score of zero means no calcium is seen in the heart. It suggests a low chance of developing a heart attack in the future.
- A score of 100-300 means moderate plaque deposits. It's associated with a relatively high risk of heart attack or other heart disease over the next three to five years.
- A score greater than 300 is a sign of very high to severe disease and heart attack risk.
- You may also receive a percentile score, which indicates your amount of calcium compared to people of the same age and sex.

Now, we know that a score of 100-400 means moderate plaque deposits with a moderately high risk of heart attack or heart disease within the next five years. My patient honestly freaked out, because this was a total shock to him. He would never have put himself in the "relatively high risk" category, especially not for having a potential heart attack within five years.

Knowing his score changed our conversation. We now had concrete information we could use to create positive changes for

---

39 Heart Scan (Coronary Calcium Scan), Mayo Clinic, https://www.mayoclinic.org/tests-procedures/heart-scan/about/pac-20384686

his health. We reflected on his diet, habits, and exercise routine. We also looked at his cholesterol panel and other lab markers. After discussing options, we created a personalized lifestyle regimen and modified his diet using the Precisionomics approach.

While it is generally not advised to check the coronary calcium score more than once every 10 years, we did recheck his other lab parameters at the six-month mark, and they had substantially improved. He lost weight and was eating a plant-focused diet, avoiding inflammatory foods, and taking gut- and heart-supportive supplements. He also began meditating and was sleeping better.

Within six months of making these changes, my patient said he felt like a "million bucks!" It's been over five years since his initial visit, and he reports continued improvements in his health and life. He says he plans on living until at least 120 years of age. Most importantly, he has not had a heart attack!

This is how knowing your health data can improve your life. This is why we use tests like the CT Coronary Calcium Scan.

What practical changes can you make as a result of having the information from this test?

For you, having the information from this test gives you a better understanding of your health, which, in turn, should empower you to have a more informed conversation with your doctor. While your doctor will make recommendations based on the data, ultimately, it's up to you to implement any necessary lifestyle changes. Having concrete data often reinforces our resolve when undergoing behavioral modifications.

Creating the best plan for you is possible because of testing like this. As a physician, this data allows us to do several things:

- We can guide medical and lifestyle changes to specifically help reduce the risk of heart disease and heart attack;

- We can understand how aggressive or intensive our interventions should be based on the score; and

- We can know if there is an imminent risk of a major event, or not.

I often say that "the only way to know, is to know."

In order to understand what types of changes might be best for you, it is important to know how your body is presently handling—and reacting to—your current way of life. Only when we have this information, such as your CT Coronary Calcium Score, can we best determine how to proceed.

CHAPTER 7

KNOWING YOUR INTERNAL BMI

The third test I recommend is the body composition test, and here's why. The body composition test affords us the opportunity to better visualize our own bodies. Your body is scanned using rapid MRI technology to measure the amount of lean tissue (muscle) and visceral adipose tissue (VAT) in your body. This test is basically a way for us to see inside the skin layer (without doing anything invasive), in a way that allows us to assess underlying risk factors based on body composition. A picture is worth a thousand words, right?

You can think of this test as measuring your internal Body Mass Index (BMI); however, body composition imaging is much more accurate. The Body Mass Index is actually just a ratio between your weight and height and is not used as often anymore on its own because of its "limited utility for predicting adverse cardiovascular outcomes."[40] It is best reserved as a population-level measurement,[41] which is to say that it is most effective when used as a data point in assessing entire populations—such as the percentage of obesity in an entire nation—which might then play a role in determining health policy.

In order to get a more accurate picture (literally) of your body than the BMI, we use body composition imaging. This test uses

---

40 Hurt RT, Kulisek C, Buchanan LA, McClave SA. The obesity epidemic: challenges, health initiatives, and implications for gastroenterologists. Gastroenterol Hepatol (N Y). 2010;6(12):780-792. https://www.ncbi.nlm.nih.gov/pmc/articles/PMC3033553/

41 Obesity and Overweight, World Health Organization, April 1, 2020, https://www.who.int/news-room/fact-sheets/detail/obesity-and-overweight

non-contrast MRI imaging, which offers no risk of radiation while providing insight into risks for conditions such as diabetes, liver disease, cancer, and cardiovascular disease. As a result, we are able to measure internal body fat in ways which offer us a much better insight into what is going on than ever before. Additionally, we are able to calculate a VAT (visceral adipose tissue) index, which measures total visceral fat then divides it by height squared.

Visceral fat is the fat that is stored within the abdominal cavity and near major organs, such as the liver, stomach, and intestines. The VAT index is connected to risk for diabetes, liver disease, and cancer. High levels of this score are the strongest body composition-related risk factor for cardiovascular events. And yes, you can be skinny and/or have normal blood work results and have a high VAT index.

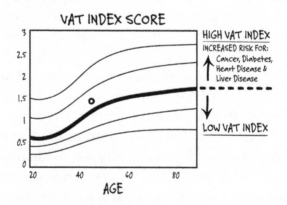

In addition to giving us a picture of visceral fat, body composition imaging also offers us insight into understanding our muscle composition. Knowing our muscle mass and its changes over time can show whether we are at risk for sarcopenia (loss of muscle as part of aging), thereby guiding our exercise practice recommendations.

Sometimes it is pertinent to do whole body imaging as well, and to use this information in conjunction with body composition imaging. Using high-end sophisticated imaging protocols can allow us to screen for cancer and neurodegenerative diseases like Alzheimer's disease in ways that we could not in the past. For the purposes of this discussion, however, we will stick to focusing on body composition imaging.

This is why Precisionomics is so important. At the end of the day we want to know what *our* risks are (and what we can do about them), not what the "potential" risk is based on epidemiologic data, or population statistics. Body composition imaging can help get us there—and when combined with whole body and brain imaging, the power of the information we collect increases, which means our ability to customize an intervention also increases.

Body composition imaging testing is a fast, non-invasive, and affordable way to understand your true fat and muscle composition, without incurring any exposure to radiation or needing an IV for contrast. Knowing a more precise ratio between your lean tissue and fatty tissue allows your doctor to more easily assess risk factors and markers for health. It also allows your doctor to have a tangible, real time marker to follow into the future to measure your progress. As we discussed, high visceral fat is associated with diabetes, liver disease, and cancer, and is the strongest body-composition associated risk factor for cardiac events.[42] In December 2018, this technology received FDA clearance, making it a game-changer in the world of Precisionomics.[43]

---

42 Bergman R.N. et al. Why visceral fat is bad: mechanisms of the metabolic syndrome. Obesity. Vol 14 supplement February 2006.

43 AMRA receives U.S. FDA clearance for AMRA® Profiler, a magnetic resonance diagnostic software application enabling non-invasive evaluation of body composition, AMRA Medical, December 11, 2018, https://www. amramedical.com/amra-receives-u-s-fda-clearance-for-amra-profiler-a-magnetic-resonance-diagnostic-software-application-enabling-non-invasive-evaluation-of-body-composition; see also AMRA Profiler Cleared by FDA for Body Composition Analysis from MRI Scans, MedGadget, January 3, 2019, https://www.medgadget.com/2019/01/amra-profiler-cleared-by-fda-for-body-composition-analysis-from-mri-scans.html

Why did I choose this test?

I really love this test because it can be incredibly eye opening, especially since it doesn't always correlate with a patient's blood markers or physical appearance. That means, for example, that you could have a normal Hgb A1c (a marker of how your body handles your blood sugar), and a reasonable BMI, and still have a high VAT score. Yes, there is such a thing as "skinny fat." How many thinner people do you know have had a heart attack? Even one, is one too many!

Here is an example of body composition scans that show two different people with the same BMI:

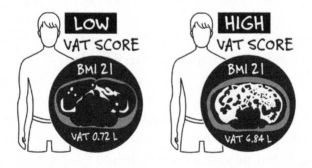

You can clearly see the difference in fatty tissue from one sample to another. When the standard tests that are performed during your annual physical exam come back as "within normal limits," this can be very misleading, giving you a false understanding of what your true risk is (see chapter 9 for more information on lab assessments). Your VAT score clears up any confusion by literally showing you—and your physician—exactly where your risk level lands.

There's an added bonus to this test, which is another reason I like it. It gives you an idea of your body's muscle composition. Knowing this may help you understand how hard you probably need to work to keep proper muscle balance, especially as you age. With this information, it will be easier to personalize your workout routines and understand what to focus on the most. If you have a personal trainer, this is information they would want to have.

What does it test?

The body composition test can identify our internal fat content and give the best evaluation for quantification of muscle groups. It has the ability to measure multiple fat and muscle biomarkers, as well as provide other body composition insights. AMRA, the Swedish corporation pioneering this technology, states:

> *Today, MRI is recognized as a golden standard for body composition analysis, enabling a more complete description of a person's body composition profile from a single examination. The precision of AMRA's healthcare technology allows for the measure of volumetric changes, and diffuse fat infiltration into muscle, unlike other less accurate techniques such as BIA (bioelectrical impedance analysis) and DXA (dual X-ray absorptiometry). [...]*

> *The body fat is divided into subcutaneous, visceral, and ectopic compartments, and each depot is given with high precision. Different muscle groups are automatically classified and the volume of each individual muscle group is obtained. Additionally, the amount of fat in any user-defined region, e.g. a muscle or an internal organ, can be calculated also for diffuse fat infiltration.*[44]

How does the test work?

While there have been other technologies along the way (such as DXA—an X-ray-based scan, which is less expensive but not remotely the same), the rapid MRI body composition scan is

---

44   The Technology, AMRA Medical, https://www.amramedical.com/technology

at the head of the pack. By scanning the entire body using this innovative technology, we are now able to see and understand small and large changes that may not be outwardly visible.

Just like a normal MRI, rapid MRI is a radiology technique that uses magnetism, radio waves, and a computer to produce images of body structures. By making it rapid, the MRI scan is better able to differentiate between the various molecules inside our body, such as water, fat, bone, and muscle.

Why is it helpful?

Because of the correlation between a high VAT index score and the incidence of disease,[45] this test gets us closer to determining your risk for a wide variety of diseases and conditions. This, in turn, helps us identify where we need to focus, since fat and muscle imbalances have been linked to chronic disease and inflammation.

Using this technology, we can gain a clearer picture of what is going on inside your body, which also allows us to identify your opportunities to decrease those risks. Historically, risks could only be addressed after an event or development of symptoms. With tests like these, we can see the potential for risks by better understanding how your unique body is functioning on multiple levels.

In order to rescue your health, you need to have the information necessary to make informed decisions. This test gives you some of the best information about your body that you can have. Combining this information with many of the other tests, such as genetics, gut microbiome testing, blood work, and other imaging, is the essence of Precisionomics and well-care.

---

45 Jensen MD, Ryan DH, Apovian CM, et al. 2013 AHA/ACC/TOS Guideline for the Management of Overweight and Obesity in Adults: A Report of the American College of Cardiology/American Heart Association Task Force on Practice Guidelines and The Obesity Society. Circulation 2014;129(25 Suppl 2):102-38.

How can the results be applied?

If you knew that you could improve your VAT index score by changing your workout routine or altering your diet, thereby reducing the risk of developing a chronic or fatal disease, you would probably do it. Knowing your ratios of fat to muscle and visceral fat to total abdominal fat can help you make more empowered decisions in your life.

Having this information can help you to:

- Develop and/or modify your diet and lifestyle regimen in a targeted manner;
- Understand what medications or supplements you might need;
- Identify what other evaluations should be done to further lower your risk factors (i.e. what other tests can we do to better understand a new risk that is now identified); and
- Direct your exercise routine more accurately.

The best part is, since this test is repeatable and something we can follow, we can actually see (quite literally) how our interventions are changing and improving your internal health.

How has this test helped someone from my practice, and why?

A 45-year-old female came to me for health optimization. After taking the standard physical-related tests and asking her various lifestyle questions, we added the body composition test to her list. The results from her lab work and office visit showed her having a BMI of 25 (normal = 18.5-24.9) and an Hgb A1c of 5.2 (normal range = 4.0-5.6), with a normal fasting blood sugar. All in all, everything seemed "normal." In this scenario, another physician might say everything was fine, but to "keep an eye on things."

However, because we added body composition imaging, we discovered that she was in the 90th percentile for her VAT index score, which is very high. While her external factors suggested that she could possibly have afforded to lose a few pounds but was generally okay, her internal evaluation suggested that there was a significant fire burning and that this fire needed to be addressed quickly before something major happened.

As a result, we put her on an aggressive lifestyle regimen, modified her diet, optimized her exercise routine, and added specific supportive treatments. Since she came to me to optimize her health, not to "keep an eye on" her health, we were able to address her unique scenario, based on her test results.

Within a month, she was losing weight, increasing her energy, and improving her sleep quality. If she had not done the body composition imaging test, she never would have known that she had a major underlying risk factor. This test allowed us to identify her hidden risk and create a personalized program that addressed her specific health issues based on the data. Ultimately, we were able to optimize her health and modify her risk factors, which would have gone unnoticed in a traditional setting with only the basic tests being performed; unnoticed, that is, until a traumatic event happened.

This is why we do these tests and practice precision medicine. This is how we stay on top of our health, rather than underneath disease.

What practical changes can you make as a result of having the information from this test?

As you have already learned, the value in doing this test lies in its ability to identify the unseen risk factors that previously weren't measurable. By knowing the ratio of our fatty tissue to our lean tissue, we are able to make better choices about our health, choices that include changes in lifestyle or more extreme interventions, if necessary.

Practically speaking, knowing your body composition can help you:

- Create more tailored and effective eating habits;
- Design a better and personalized exercise routine for your body;
- Engage in more focused conversations with your healthcare providers; and
- Intervene earlier in high-risk situations, thereby requiring less invasive procedures or solutions.

It may seem like each of these tests result in the same suggestions, and there's a reason for that. Ultimately, lifestyle and genetics are two of the key factors on which our good health depends. Most helpful interventions will address both of these elements by creating a lifestyle plan that is specific to your body's genetics. That can include behavioral changes (like food choices, habits, and exercise) and supportive changes (like supplements and medications), among others we have already reviewed in this book.

Knowing your body composition helps you make better and more targeted choices in your behavioral, supportive, and physical decisions, which often leads to optimized health.

CHAPTER 8

Nutritional Genomics

My fourth recommended test is a nutritional genomics test. We are only starting to understand the importance of nutritional genomics and the role it plays in our overall health. This is an area of study that is continually evolving as researchers look at both the role of nutrition on the human genome and the individual relationship between specific foods and specific genes.

What if you could know that any and all dairy would cause an adverse reaction in your system because of a gene you carry? Or, what if you could know it's only the lactose or the protein casein that is detrimental to your well-being? Would this change the way you eat? Could it explain a chronic symptom you have had for as long as you can remember?

Consider this explanation from molecular nutritionist Colleen Fogarty Draper:

> "Nutritional genomics is the scientific study of the impact of gene polymorphisms on the body's propensity for disease and functional imbalances and nutritional requirements; and the impact of food, nutrients, and related holistic aspects of human lifestyle on gene expression; which also affects gene regulation, transcription, early phase protein production, and intermediary markers of metabolism expressed by the metabolome. As this informative

area of science progresses, the nutritional genomics term will increasingly encompass nutritional systems biology, including all of the "omics" sciences as they relate to nutrition, lifestyle, life experiences, and other related aspects of the environment that contribute to an individual's well-being."[46]

This quote is an all-encompassing way of saying that although the research is ongoing, this is an important test to consider. This is not a food sensitivity test. It goes well beyond the standard "food allergy or sensitivity" tests, because it looks at your blueprint—your genes—to get specific answers on what and how to eat.

While whole genome testing is valuable, it may not be affordable for everyone. If whole genome sequencing (or whole exome sequencing) isn't feasible, then nutritional genomics is a worthwhile alternative. Yes, there are limitations to testing only certain sets of genes, but when you choose this option, you do so understanding and acknowledging those limitations from the start. The important thing is to do the most you can with the resources you have to gather the information you can acquire.

A nutritional genomics test can provide you with a solid starting point from which to optimize your health. In fact, studies have shown that dietary changes are more sustainable and successful when they are derived from the tailored approach available by conducting a nutritional genomics test, instead of suggesting one of the more common one-size-fits-all dietary approaches so prevalent in the world today.[47]

Of course, there are many applications for this test, from dietary modifications to supplementation and beyond. What seems to matter even more, however, is the role this test plays in motivation

---

46 Colleen Fogarty Draper, Nutrigenomics and Nutrigenetics in Functional Food and Personalized Nutrition, CRC Press – Taylor and Francis Group (2016), chapter 18, p. 347.

47 Nielsen DE, El-Sohemy A. Disclosure of genetic information and change in dietary intake: a randomized controlled trial. PLoS One. 2014;9(11):e112665.

when it comes to behavior modification. As researchers in a 2020 study on nutritional genomics testing concluded:

> *"...a systematic review of DTC [Direct To Consumer] testing and its effects on health behaviors concluded that, while the effect is modest, commercial DTC tests do motivate improvements in exercise and dietary habits and encourage individuals to give up smoking. These results suggest that information obtained from a DTC genetic test does impact health behavior, particularly dietary behavior, in a considerable proportion of users."*[48]

So, if you're looking for ways to increase your motivation to change—or if you've struggled with staying motivated in the past—this test could be a game-changer for you. Knowing your body's specific needs is more effective at optimizing your health than making your best guess based on everyone else around you.

Nutritional genomics is an important tool that can offer us insight into what our bodies are missing and might need. If, for example, we can discover that our risk for Vitamin C deficiency is greater than that of the average person, then we can make a positive intervention to address that risk before it becomes a problem. Insight in this manner can help us make lifestyle modifications that are more in alignment with our personal disposition.

It's not just limited to vitamins and nutrition, either. For example, if you knew your genetic predisposition to how you might be programmed to excel in athletics, you could plan your workout routines accordingly and understand what you need to do in order to succeed in optimizing your health. Alternatively, if you knew you were among the population at increased risk for high blood pressure and/or heart attack from eating too much salt or

---

48 Guest, N., Jamnik, J., Garcia-Bailo, B., Nielsen, D.E., El-Sohemy, A. (2020). Applying Genomics for Personalized Nutrition in Clinical Practice. In G. E. Mullin, M. M. Singh, A. M. Parian, & J. Clarke (Eds.), Integrative Gastroenterology (2nd ed., p.574). Oxford University Press.

drinking too much caffeine, you could make a more informed decision in your food choices.

Understanding your genetic risks for these things can help you make simple lifestyle modifications that could literally be lifesaving down the road.

Nutritional Deficiencies

Depending on where you live and your age range, most annual exams include blood work that measures certain vitamin levels. Testing for vitamin levels helps us understand if you need vitamin supplements to support your body's processes. These nutrients act as cofactors in numerous reactions that occur in our body, and we need them for many different reasons. If we are running low on something and we discover it, supplementing that deficiency could mean the difference between our engine running at the best of its ability or barely running at all.

Gathering this information helps us understand where we can modify or improve the diet—which, in turn, can positively impact quality of life. While I run regular blood level tests such as B12, RBC folate, Magnesium, Vitamin D, and others, I also like to conduct a more focused test when the situation calls for it and to include micronutrients.

Micronutrient testing measures the function of the nutritional components—including vitamins, antioxidants, minerals, and amino acids—within our white blood cells. Analyzing these white blood cells can give a more accurate analysis of a body's deficiencies. So, when a patient's symptoms call for more detailed information, I'll opt for this test. Again, it's all about tailoring the test to the situation and gathering as much data as you can in order to make more informed decisions about your health and well-being. These tests can certainly be complementary to someone's evaluation when we are running a nutritional genomics panel.

Broader Implications

There are broader implications for nutritional genomics, as well. Beyond knowing your personal nutritional genetic profile, we can expand upon that information to make decisions that could change the healthcare landscape as a whole. As one set of researchers has put it:

> "The public health significance of nutrigenomic testing lies within its potential use as an early detection method to identify individual susceptibility and population subgroups propensities based on responses to various dietary components and genetic predisposition to a spectrum of diseases."[49]

Truly, knowing our nutritional genomics has so many positive implications on our health, both individually and as a society. For that reason alone, this test is in my top five. We are able to learn a lot from our genetics that can positively impact how we approach nutrition. This is what nutritional genomics is.

Why did I choose this test?

I chose this test because it's more financially accessible for many people. Doing whole exome or whole genome sequencing is not always financially possible. However, that does not mean that you cannot do *any* genetic testing to get meaningful information about your health and what nutritional choices to make. The nutritional genomics panel costs approximately $300 and is a more affordable way to gather impactful information regarding the propensity for nutrient deficiencies.

Additionally, we can get information from this test that can help guide your exercise prescription (i.e. how you should exercise

---

49   Elizabeth H Marchlewicz, Karen E Peterson, and Gilbert S Omenn, Public Health Context for Nutrigenomics and Personalized Nutrition, Chapter 20, page 379.

and what exercises you might excel in). This test is a simple way to gather a lot of meaningful information at an affordable price.

What does it test?

A nutritional genomics panel looks at a variety of SNPs (single nucleotide polymorphisms) to receive insight into how your body is programmed. What are Single Nucleotide Polymorphisms? Dr. Francis S. Collins, the physician and geneticist who has led both the Human Genome Project and the National Institutes of Health, has a really wonderful explanation:

> *"[SNPs] are the places in the genome where people differ. In about one out of every 1,000 letters of the code you'll run into one of these where I might have a C and you might have a T, and we'd call that a SNP. Most SNPs don't do very much, 'cause they're in a part of the genome that doesn't have a critical function. But some of them confer a risk of disease like diabetes or heart disease, and those are of intense current interest because of what they teach us about why those diseases happen."*[50]

There are numerous companies that do this kind of testing, and each one looks for a variety of genes that are pertinent to aspects of nutrition. Essentially, what we are trying to understand is how your unique body is programmed. That's the bottom line for these tests, and the implications are nearly endless.

For example, knowing if you have an MTHFR (Methylenetetra-hydrofolate reductase) mutation will help you understand what the potential for your folate status may be. We know that there are links between MTHFR and various diseases, such as tumors, as well as cardiovascular and neurologic diseases. We also know that "as both DNA methylation and folate are important in mental

---

50   Single Nucleotide Polymorphisms (SNPs), National Human Genome Research Institute, https://www.genome.gov/genetics-glossary/Single-Nucleotide-Polymorphisms

health, reduction of MTHFR activity or folate deficiency have been associated with an onset of several psychiatric diseases, schizophrenia, bipolar disorder, depression, autism, and ADHD."[51] If you knew you were at risk for an increase in disease due to a nutritional gene mutation, you'd want to do something about it, wouldn't you?

Having this specific information can guide our interventions differently, which can improve our chances for positive outcomes. Here's a really simple example of what that could look like:

> Let's say one person has a gene mutation that suggests that they may need higher amounts of Vitamin C in order to get the same total amount in their bloodstream as someone who does not have the gene mutation. This might suggest that if the two people eat the same orange, the person with the gene mutation may be less likely to have the proper Vitamin C response in the body compared to the other person. In effect, he/she may need to eat more oranges to get the same impact as the person without the gene mutation.

Of course, this is just an example for the purposes of demonstrating some of the simplest ways we can use the data from this test. Whether you need one or more oranges is not based on any study. I'm just making a simple analogy so you can understand the importance of this test and how having this information can help you rescue your health.

Additionally, there are some genes that pertain to exercise, which may give us insight into whether your body would excel in strength-based exercise or endurance-based exercise. With this information, we can also understand if you are more likely to have improvement in insulin levels with exercise. We can also understand if you are at increased risk of an Achilles tendon injury. Cool, right?

---

51 Wan L, Li Y, Zhang Z, Sun Z, He Y, Li R. Methylenetetrahydrofolate reductase and psychiatric diseases. Transl Psychiatry. 2018;8(1):242. Published 2018 Nov 5. https://www.ncbi.nlm.nih.gov/pmc/articles/PMC6218441/

More importantly, perhaps, the information from this test can help us understand if you are more likely to have a heart attack from drinking more than two cups of coffee, or if you are more likely to develop high blood pressure from eating more than 1500mg of salt in your daily diet.

I think at this point you can see the value in these kinds of nutritional genomic tests, because they can give you insight into dietary habits that you would never have known without checking how you, personally, are programmed.

How does the test work?

Many of these tests are simple. They are either a saliva (spit) sample or a buccal swab (swabbing the inside of your cheek). They usually take a minute or two to collect, after which they are preserved in a solution to be transported without degrading. The lab then specifically analyzes the sample to let you know what gene mutations you do or do not have.

Why is it helpful?

Understanding your nutritional genomics—especially your specific mutations—is helpful because it allows us to gain a deeper and more detailed understanding into how we can optimize our health, through:

- identifying what foods we should eat more of to prevent nutrient deficiencies;
- creating more tailored exercise routines so we can excel in weight loss;
- understanding how best to manage our calorie intake in order to lose weight;
- knowing if we are at risk for issues with gluten and/or dairy;

- modifying our behaviors to reduce the risk of heart disease and many other chronic diseases; and

- planning our macros (how much fat, protein, and carbohydrates we should eat) to help our body function at the optimal level.

How can the results be applied?

The Precisionomics approach to nutrition would include taking this type of information, looking at food sensitivities, personal preferences, socio-economic situations, the gut microbiome, and any particular symptoms someone might have, and then making recommendations on how to start modifying your diet and lifestyle with all of that in mind. With this information, we can also make recommendations on how to exercise (what type and at what intensity) and give information to your trainer that can help you excel, while also reducing the chance for injury.

Knowledge is power. If you know that your risk of having a heart attack increases significantly from drinking a pot of coffee every day, or that you have a gene mutation that increases your risk of psychiatric disease, you now have the information to make a change, and improve your health outcomes.

How has this test helped someone from my practice, and why?

A good, simple, and impactful example from my practice is that of a patient who wanted to know how to optimize their diet. They had been on a vegan diet and were experiencing some fatigue and depression. We conducted the nutritional genomic panel, and they were found to have a genetic mutation that would increase their risk of B12 deficiency. Of course, we also checked B12 levels to see what the status was at the time. Not surprisingly, the patient was found to be profoundly B12 deficient.

As a result, we were able to make a tailored intervention that included a discussion on what the best diet may be for them in the long run and how to include sources of B12 in their diet.[52] Many of the patient's complaints regarding fatigue and depression started to improve dramatically with the addition of B12. This opened the door to a deeper conversation about their diet choice, what they really wanted to pursue, and most importantly, why.

There are many reasons why someone would like to pursue a particular diet over another. Knowing your nutritional genomics can help you make a more informed decision about your diet. There is no problem in choosing virtually any diet, especially when you understand how a particular eating style might impact your health in a variety of ways. Consulting with your doctor to strategize ways around obstacles is the key to optimizing your health.

A note about diet

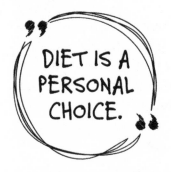

As a physician, I am not pro-vegan or pro- any particular diet. To me, "diet" is actually a bad word. There is no universal diet that works for everyone. What matters is that you know how your body is programmed. What you want, and what you might think is good for you, might not actually be the best for you. By understanding this, we can make an educated decision on what *your eating style* (not diet) should be. The only eating style that is important, is the one that works for YOU!

---

52 The A List of B12 Foods, Harvard Health Publishing, Harvard Medical School, https://www.health.harvard.edu/staying-healthy/the-a-list-of-b12-foods

What practical changes can you make as a result of having the data from this test?

By understanding your unique nutritional genetic makeup, you can create opportunities to optimize your health and well-being that include:

- Personalized exercise habits for better results;
- Increased nutritional balance and easier-to-maintain eating habits;
- Better weight management;
- Decreased injury risk; and
- Lowered risk of nutritional deficiency and food intolerance.

Not only will you have the information you need to make better dietary decisions, you will also have the information you need to increase your cardiometabolic health and tailor your exercise program to meet your specific needs. This test is a win-win when it comes to lifestyle changes.

CHAPTER 9

LAB ASSESSMENTS

My final 'top five' test is the one you are already most likely to have had done: a full slate of basic lab assessments. Ideally, we are all having a physical examination every year, and part of that includes having our lab work done. Starting this process early (in your 30s) gives you a strong baseline from which we can identify any variations over time.

A lab assessment typically includes blood work that looks at: complete blood count, comprehensive metabolic panel, hormone levels, cholesterol levels, and diabetes (blood sugar) factors, among other indicators. Beyond these basics, we can also look at: inflammation levels, nutrient levels, Omega 3 levels, and vitamin levels, to name a few. This is a standard of care that is usually covered by insurance and should be the minimum we do on at least an annual basis to understand our own health.

As we've clearly established, you can look healthy on the outside, but the internal numbers may tell a very different story—or vice versa. As I've already mentioned, there are some standard tests that every physician typically includes in their lab assessments. In my practice, I almost always include a test for inflammation levels, because inflammation is one of the underlying hidden causes of ill health.

Having a conversation with your physician to address your concerns is the best place to start. If you're having baseline tests completed in your 30s, for example, you might want to do a broader range of tests simply to have that benchmark information for the future.

Why did I choose this test?

Basic lab assessments are the simplest to do and should be entirely covered by insurance. This means that there should be no barriers to performing these assessments on a regular basis, outside of any copay obligations you may have. These types of tests give us a preliminary idea of how your body is working. It is one thing to look at the various genetics of things or to see what the gut microbiome is doing, but it is imperative that we gain some insight into what the result of all this is. Basic lab tests are a way of understanding what is actually happening on the inside. To put it more clearly, these lab assessments tell you how your body is functioning on a daily basis, in real time, answering such questions as:

- How is your body managing blood sugar?
- Do you have significant inflammation in the body?
- What are your actual vitamin and nutrient levels?
- How are your hormones doing?
- How are your kidneys and liver working?
- Are you anemic?

Having these answers can help us understand what your body might need *right now,* giving us a really good place to start. This will help us optimize things in the short term that will then help with your long-term outcomes. I often say we have to get you there to keep you there. If we do not know what some of the obstacles are then we won't know what the best initial direction should be.

Most importantly, these are such simple tests that we can use them on an ongoing basis to follow your progress. They will let us know if what we are doing is helping so that we can shift gears if needed to ensure we keep steering you in the right direction.

What does it test?

There are a wide variety of tests that various practitioners might consider "basic," but I think that doing several of the below tests are a reasonable place to start. One could certainly do more (or less!), but the point is to do at least a few of these tests so we can see your body's current state of affairs. Since so many tests can fall under the category "Lab Assessments," I will try to break down the importance of why we do these tests, and what tests I prefer.

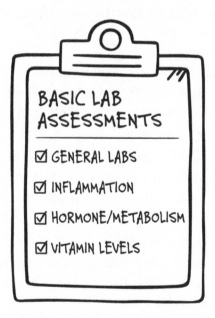

General Labs - Both a CBC and CMP are done to get a broad overview of your body's overall functioning. These tests tell us if there are any red flags that require further investigation.

- CBC (complete blood count): looks at the levels of white blood cells, hemoglobin, platelets, and other parameters

- CMP (comprehensive metabolic panel): looks at your electrolytes, kidney, and liver function

Inflammation - There are myriad blood tests that can offer insight into any inflammation that could be occurring in the heart or vascular system. The results from any one of these tests allow us to understand if there is something brewing in the background, something unseen and, hopefully, preventable. Testing for inflammatory markers is a bit like doing an initial survey on an archeological dig. It helps us understand if there's an area we need to focus on and dig further. Inflammatory markers can push us toward identifying the source of a problem before it becomes a problem.

- ESR (Erythrocyte Sedimentation Rate or Sed Rate) and hs-CRP (High Sensitivity C-Reactive Protein): used to detect non-specific markers of inflammation in the body

- Advanced Cardiac Markers: used to look more closely at the different kinds of lipids you have, as well as particle numbers (and sizes) of these lipids, and give us an idea regarding what level of severity your heart problem might be

- ox-LDL (Oxidized Low-density Lipoprotein): used to detect metabolic syndrome and cardiovascular disease because it contributes to plaque formation and progression in the heart

- ADMA (asymmetric dimethylarginine): used to detect damage to the endothelium, or the inner lining of blood vessels

- Myeloperoxidase (MPO): used to help us understand the degree of inflammation at the level of the arterial wall

- NMR lipid panel (Nuclear Magnetic Resonance lipid panel): used to measure LDL particles in both number and size, as well as HDL and VLDL subclasses

- TMAO* (Trimethylamine N-Oxide; a blood marker of gut imbalance that can offer risk for heart disease): used to detect a metabolite from gut bacteria that is associated with increased risk of heart attack or stroke

- Omega 3 levels and Omega 6:3 ratio: used to measure the ratio of fatty acids in your bloodstream

- Homocysteine: an independent risk factor for cardiovascular disease which can also help in detection of deficiencies of B vitamins

*A brief science lesson: TMA (Trimethylamine) is a metabolite or product made by bacteria in the gut microbiome. It goes to the liver and is converted to TMAO and has a direct correlation with increased risk of heart disease. From the National Institutes of Health:

> *In humans, recent clinical studies evidence a positive correlation between elevated plasma levels of TMAO and an increased risk for major adverse cardiovascular events. A direct correlation between increased TMAO levels and neurological disorders has been also hypothesized.*[53]

Hormone/Metabolism - These tests give us an insight into key areas of your body's hormone function (and dysfunction) as well as metabolism.

- Thyroid function tests, including thyroid antibodies for Hashimoto's disease: used to measure the level of thyroid hormones in the blood

53 Janeiro MH, Ramírez MJ, Milagro FI, Martínez JA, Solas M. Implication of Trimethylamine N-Oxide (TMAO) in Disease: Potential Biomarker or New Therapeutic Target. Nutrients. 2018;10(10):1398. Published 2018 Oct 1. https://www.ncbi.nlm.nih.gov/pmc/articles/PMC6213249/

- Cortisol: used to measure levels of cortisol in the blood, which can indicate problems with the adrenal glands or pituitary gland (this is known as the stress hormone)
- Hgb A1c: used to measure the *average* blood sugar levels in your blood over the previous three months
- Female Hormone panels: used to measure reproductive abilities and female-specific hormones in women
- Male Hormone panels: used to measure testosterone and other male-specific hormones in men

Vitamins levels

- Vitamin D: deficiency of Vitamin D can be associated with bone weakness, bone malformation, calcium metabolism, and a whole host of other things, including a suboptimal immune system
- B12 and RBC folate: measured within the liquid portion of the blood, these nutrients are needed for healthy functioning, including by creating red blood cells and supporting RNA and DNA to help build cells
- Zinc: Zinc is an essential element in the body for numerous systems, particularly the immune system
- Coenzyme Q10 levels: deficient CoQ10 levels are associated with conditions that affect the heart; deficiencies can also lead to mitochondrial dysfunction

How does the test work?

These are simple blood tests. Your doctor can prescribe these tests for you, which are conducted at his/her regular lab or through a mobile phlebotomist (someone trained to draw blood) who can come to you if needed. Based on the tests requested, it's most likely that a few tubes of blood will be drawn. Making sure you are properly hydrated before the tests are conducted will make it easier. Also, be sure to check with your physician on whether a test requires you to be fasting (not having eaten within 12 hours, or sometimes more), or off of your Omega 3 supplement 24 hours prior. Within about a week or less, the results are sent to your doctor for review.

Why is it helpful?

Basic lab assessments can help stratify risk and give us both a starting point and a general direction. In short, they help us prioritize where we should put our focus to have the greatest impact on improving our health and well-being. They let us know many things, such as:

- if there is protoplasm for heart disease;
- whether there is an imbalance of cholesterol;
- how much inflammation is in your body;
- if there are any nutrient deficiencies; and
- if there are any hormone imbalances.

The lab results are a current snapshot of how your body is doing, how it is coping, and where it is having difficulty or is stressed. We can then use this information to make the best decisions in regard to any interventions.

These lab assessments go hand-in-hand with the other tests I've already mentioned. While it is important to know your genetic risks and other risk factors, it is also important to have an understanding of what is happening right now and in what order we should proceed with any changes.

How can the results be applied?

Your doctor can use these results to understand if you need certain treatments or medications. They can also help you formulate the best lifestyle regimen for you. After that, these tests can be used as markers of progress. Being able to see physical changes in the numbers is one of the greatest motivating factors on our journey to good health. When we know that the behavioral changes we have made are producing results, we are more likely to stick with them for the long haul.

How has this test helped someone from my practice, and why?

One example that comes to mind is a patient who outwardly appeared fit and was actually resistant to even checking cholesterol and inflammation levels because he believed it was pointless. He thought there was no way he could have any issues, since he presumed himself to be healthy based on his appearance.

There are plenty of people like this. Just because a person may be skinny or appear fit does not mean that their cholesterol and inflammation levels are low. How many people have you known or seen that had heart attacks that were not overweight or diabetic? Even trainers and athletes can suffer from a heart attack or a stroke. Just because someone looks good, doesn't mean the numbers match, and vice versa.

Back to my patient. Ultimately, he agreed to conduct the basic lab assessments. When we received the results, we discovered three things: 1) his cholesterol panel was completely off, 2) he had severe Vitamin D deficiency, and 3) he had a very high TMAO level (Trimethylamine N-Oxide).

Knowing his results, we discussed his lifestyle, including his eating habits. He understood that his meat-based diet might not be the best for him (increased levels of TMAO are found to be associated with diets heavy in red meats, dairy, and eggs), and his hope was to stay off of cholesterol medication. So, we focused on putting together a meaningful eating style and lifestyle plan based on his lab results that would show us how his body was functioning in real-time. Plus, in order to increase his Vitamin D levels, we added supplementation as well as more outdoor exercise.

Upon the next round of testing, we saw results. By diversifying his diet, his TMAO level dropped and his cholesterol panel improved. We also noted that his inflammatory markers—which were slightly elevated— had normalized.

The bottom line is that we were able to put out a smoldering fire before it became a full-blown inferno by doing some basic lab assessments, at no cost to him outside of his insurance copay. Even better, with regular testing we can continue to monitor and modify things, ensuring that the fire doesn't start again.

What practical changes can you make as a result of having the information from this test?

Lab assessments are the minimum we should be doing on an annual basis to understand our health and how well (or poorly) our body is functioning. Just a few of the things we can do with these tests:

- We can modify eating style and exercise habits.
- We can choose what supplements are best for someone.
- We can follow this data to look for markers of progress.
- We can understand risk for chronic disease and inflammatory problems even before an actual problem surfaces (like a heart attack, developing diabetes, or having an autoimmune disease for example).

As a result of this information, we can make meaningful modifications that usually result in an immediate impact.

Rescuing your health doesn't have to require sweeping change like going from eating a variety of meats to being a vegan, or from walking a bit every day to running a marathon. No, rescuing your health means that you take the time to get the health data you need to make more informed choices for your *own* body in meaningful ways, and then implementing them.

Now that we have the technology and science to gather data more efficiently and economically, the only thing missing is you. What could you do with a little more information about how *your* body works? How could it change your life for the better?

We have covered a lot of ground in Part I of this book, and I hope you found the information inspiring and informative—enough so that you have started to make a list of questions to bring to your physician so that you can get started on your own path of optimizing your longevity and well-being. To help you in that journey, we have compiled a set of resources in the Appendix that you can use.

In the next section, I share the personal stories of various patients I have worked with over the years who took those first steps toward rescuing their health. Like so many others, at first they didn't know where to start. Often, they were frustrated from either a lack of accurate diagnoses or a chronic condition that was only being managed just enough to remain tolerable without ever improving.

These individuals wanted a different way—a new way—to look at and be in relationship with their body, and they found it in the precision medicine approach. They found it in Precisionomics. Hopefully, you will too.

PART II:

HOW PERSONALIZED MEDICINE CAN HELP YOU RESCUE YOUR HEALTH

CHAPTER 10

Why Personalized Information is So Important

In the first half of this book, we addressed the science behind the medicine. Specifically, we looked at the body and all its systems as well as the various advances in science and technology that have allowed for the creation of precision medicine. Having all of this information is great, but it doesn't help us if we don't know how to use it.

One of the reasons I became a physician was to help people improve their quality of life. Theoretically, that meant managing symptoms and treating disease. As I went through medical school, I learned that while we may hope for a cure, we spend most of our days and expertise working with our patients to address the manifestation of their disease, better known as their discomfort. They come to us because something has already gone "wrong," and we need to take care of their symptoms first.

While this is an important part of medicine—I can't imagine a world without the interventions we currently use to treat an array of ailments—I wanted to learn how to stay ahead of disease, not behind it.

Health is not a destination. There isn't a point at which you've "arrived" and no longer have to do anything else to stay healthy. Not in today's world, at least. In fact, as I was writing this book, I was reminded of the small tear in my shoulder. It flares up every now and then, which serves as a reminder to me that there are things I can do to help myself on a regular basis.

Good health is the sum of all the choices you make day after day after day. It's cumulative. It's about participating in your life and investing in ownership of your body. That's why this book is called *Rescue Your Health.* You are your own rescuer. You have to invest in your health if you want to stay strong and resilient.

You don't buy a house or a car and then stop taking care of it. If you did, you'd end up with a lot of problems in a short period of time. So, why would you rescue your health by only doing the minimum, such as getting an annual physical and nothing more? Or handing everything over to chance or someone else to manage? You wouldn't. At least, I hope you wouldn't. But if you did, just like my shoulder, you would get little reminders every now and then that good health isn't a "one-and-done" endeavor.

Every health-related situation has some measure of a solution. Often, there is a crossover in what solutions are applied. For example, a modification in what food a patient eats might serve as the same suggestion for both someone with chronic allergies and someone with heart disease.

As you now know, precision medicine allows us to tailor interventions to the specific needs of the individual. However, over the course of my career, I have seen patterns and similarities in how symptoms present across a spectrum of patients. Therefore, in order to make this information easier to apply in your own life, I have identified some specific patient "types" using examples from my practice.

Perhaps you will see yourself in one of these patient stories. Or, maybe you will relate to different aspects from a few of them. If so,

I hope it will give you some ideas of what you could do to decrease your symptoms and optimize your health. That is the goal, after all.

Without good health, life becomes increasingly more challenging. Of course, the best approach would be to do your own testing to learn the specifics about your body and what it needs. However, I know that's not realistic for everyone. So, I included these examples to help give you a good starting point to understand what's possible and then discuss it with your doctor. I also think it might be helpful to know how I approach each new patient, and what I ask them to bring to our first appointment together. As such, I have compiled a few items in the Appendix to help you take the first step on your journey to rescuing your health. So now let's look at how I start with anybody new to my clinic.

When a new patient arrives at my clinic, we always start with a comprehensive history. This includes any previous diagnoses and a list of current symptoms. I will also review all the prior test results they have had. From there, I can make the best decisions based on the patient's budget and needs, focusing on the tests that will have the greatest impact and give us the information we need to make positive changes. Of course, when we are trying to do a deep search for the cause of your symptoms or problems, we take as comprehensive an approach as possible to evaluate as many of the major factors as possible that can influence health.

Thankfully, these tests can be personalized if there is a specific problem, and we can do more if we need to, as you will see in the upcoming chapters. Not everyone will need body imaging or whole genome sequencing. We do our best to get as much information as possible, within the scope of what's available and what's needed. If we only did one or two tests based on previous diagnoses or reported symptoms, we might miss something. Even though symptoms can be similar in two different individuals, the root cause may vary.

As you will see, each of the following chapters highlights a patient story that represents one of the "types" I mentioned above.[54] These broader categories are often related to specific body systems, and I have compiled them to help make it easier to understand how symptoms can show up based on the system they most affect.

In short, these are the most common categories of symptoms or "types" of patient issues that I see in my practice:

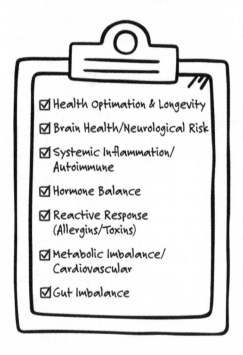

While this is not an extensive list of patient complaints, it's a good starting point for us. As you read the following chapters and get to know some of my patients, take note of your own situation. Perhaps you will identify with aspects of John's story, who wanted

54   Names and identifying information have been changed for confidentiality

to optimize his health and longevity. Or, perhaps you will relate to Jennifer who simply "didn't feel like she used to."

Whenever you find yourself identifying with one of the individuals in the upcoming chapters, it would be a good idea to write it down. This will give you a good base from which to start a conversation with your doctor. While the chapters are not meant to diagnose or treat you (I can't do that from within the pages of a book), they are meant to inspire you. My hope is that you will take note of something and use it to create positive change in your life. Of course, you should always check with your own doctor first, before embarking on any specific modifications, especially if they involve medicine or supplements.

CHAPTER 11

Optimizing Your Health and Longevity

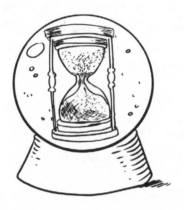

When I think about "rescuing your health," I think about this patient profile. This is all of us. Who wouldn't want to increase their years, especially if their health is optimized? One of the most common things I hear on a regular basis is: "I don't feel particularly ill, but I know I want to feel better, and I don't know where to start."

John came to me with this exact situation. With a busy career and a young family, he had a desire to know more so he could make more informed decisions. While there was no specific complaint he could identify, he had just turned 40 and had started to think about his own mortality, which made him a little nervous with a young family at home.

John wanted to be able to work hard, have fun, enjoy life, and provide a great environment for his wife and kids. Without any diagnosis of disease, John wasn't sick or experiencing symptoms. He simply had a feeling that maybe he should ask some questions.

John is the "everyman" or "everywoman." He's probably what someone might consider "average," but average isn't necessarily healthy. And, without any concrete diagnoses, he's arguably better than most.

As humans, we have intuition, and that intuition can only be ignored for so long. In John's case, he probably knew for over a decade that he wanted to make some changes, he just didn't know the three W's to help get him started: Where, What, and Why.

- Where do I begin?
- What should I (specifically) focus on?
- Why should I make changes?

While John wasn't specifically asking these three questions, he knew enough to know that he should probably start looking at his health a bit more closely.

John's childhood was "normal," for all intents and purposes. He grew up happy with very few problems. In fact, there was nothing remarkable about his history until he mentioned getting sick around age eight and having to stay out of school for a few months.

After he recovered, his life continued. He played sports, had friends, and rarely was sick again, citing only a handful of illnesses that required antibiotic treatment. John ate home-cooked meals every day, and enjoyed a full life throughout his teenage years. The only trauma he could identify from his youth was his parents' divorce.

His childhood seemed to mirror most of his adulthood, in that there was nothing glaring to "fix" or address. Everything was steady with no identifiable issues or problems. In fact, John exercised regularly and ate well until he was in his early 30s.

While he didn't classify himself as "unhealthy," he identified his early 30s as the point at which things started to change, and not for the better. His growing career and an unexpected injury meant he stepped away from exercising regularly. It also impacted his eating habits, with fast food now on the menu. After about a decade of these lifestyle changes, he started to feel like it was time to reassess.

That was when he called me.

Even though he had made some modifications on his own, such as switching to a more plant-based diet, he knew he needed more information in order to make better decisions and really understand what his specific risks were so that he could make specific changes in his life.

In many ways, John is someone we all know. Young, seemingly healthy, with a good career, a happy (also young) family, and very little extra time to prioritize himself. Even though he owned home workout equipment, he rarely used it. Between the demands of work and family his stress levels were increasing over time.

Additionally, his own parents were aging, which required more of him and added to his increasing stress. With a diminished amount of available time, socializing was one of the first things to go. Even though he said he didn't mind that shift—his family and work made him very happy—being able to socialize with a peer group is known to be beneficial to our overall health.

During our appointment, John mentioned he had a friend who got a clean bill of health from his primary care doctor and had a major heart attack several months later. Understandably, John didn't want that to be him. So, with the increase in stress and the decrease in available time to do anything about it, he made the decision to learn more about his individual health and where he could focus his energy to greatest effect.

For someone like John—or all of us—it could be as simple as saying, "eat healthier and exercise more," which is pretty common advice. However, when you want to optimize your health, a generic solution like that isn't really an answer.

John let me know that he wanted to lose about 10-20 pounds and that his cholesterol was slightly higher than he would like. Again, these are more general goals that many people have without any additional specific data. In John's case, there were no other outstanding markers or measurements that he could report.

So, my focus was on helping John to create and prioritize specific goals that we could identify by customizing his tests. At his request, and my suggestion, we took a comprehensive approach. He was "all in" and at the perfect age to get a baseline understanding of his health. The more we could learn now, the better off he would be for the future.

Looking back, I think John was both curious and excited—though perhaps a little concerned—to learn how his body was functioning. We completed a full panel of tests that included:

- body composition imaging
- whole body
  and brain MRI
- cardiac MRI
- CT coronary
  calcium score
- whole genome sequencing
- micronutrient testing
- food sensitivity testing

- evaluation for toxins
- evaluation for advanced cardiac markers
- evaluation of the microbiome
- evaluation of his telomere length
- test for leaky gut

Once we had the results, we knew exactly where to start. Like most patients I work with, we always focus on their personal goals. For John:

- He wanted to live healthier for longer.
- He wanted to be able to see his young kids grow up and become his friends.
- He wanted to be able to keep working until he no longer wanted to work anymore, not because his body couldn't handle it.
- He wanted to grow old with his wife and enjoy a comfortable retirement together.
- He wanted to improve his longevity by focusing on his health now.

While John had no specific complaints, he knew that he wanted to make meaningful changes now that would carry him forward well into the future.

Most of his key results came back as "normal" or "insignificant." This was great news! It meant that we could target specific areas to positively impact his health and his longevity.

Interestingly, one of the most important findings was that he carried a gene mutation for Alzheimer's disease, the APOE gene. This means that he statistically had a 3-fold increased risk of developing Alzheimer's disease during his lifetime and a 22% increased risk of heart disease.

While this could be concerning to some, the highly specialized heart and brain imaging tests we did came out perfect. We were able to reassure him that there was no immediate threat to his health and that if we worked together to eliminate factors that could drive this risk and we continually followed his progress, we could do our best to ensure that his genes were not his destiny and that his goals in life were still possible.

John was so happy to know that he had this gene at this early age because now he had the chance to do the best he could to prevent getting the condition, or at least greatly postpone when he might develop any issues. He realized that he did not have to be a statistic and that he was not going to fall into the category of the general population's risk for Alzheimer's disease. We had enough tools in our toolbox now to reduce his personal risk, which is the goal.

The test results gave us the information we needed to focus on the changes that would make the biggest difference in John's life, knowing that he would continue to live a very busy life with his career and family.

We prioritized several specific areas, using the tests we conducted to help us hone in on key areas that could use some improving. By knowing his risk factors, I was able to recommend the following:

- Specific supplement suggestions that would work with his body and support the very few and slight imbalances that resulted from the testing
- Diet modifications that included cycling between three different focused approaches by month, to make life easier for him and his family
- Environmental changes to mitigate the toxin exposure that showed up on his test results, such as having his home tested for mold and changing his water filtration system

- Apps, tools, and behavior changes to improve his quality of sleep
- Simple daily practices that would be accessible to him in order to reduce his stress, including time-limited practices, such as setting a daily intention Incorporating scheduled "family fun time," "date night," and "social activities" into his monthly schedule in order to maintain a healthier balance in his life
- Ongoing support with specific, hand-picked supplements for detoxification, reducing inflammation, improving mitochondrial health, and optimizing gut health. Some of the things we included in his regimen were liposomal glutathione, B vitamins, Curcumin, Vitamin D, Fish oil, Nicotinamide Riboside, probiotics, L-glutamine, Vitamin C, Vitamin K2, Digestive enzymes, Resveratrol, and prebiotics

I was also able to make John aware of his elevated risk for injury in his feet when exercising, and suggest strength training as his primary focus for exercise, with cardiovascular workouts being supplementary—including a recommendation for a target amount of time spent exercising each week. I was even able to explain to John why certain types of alcohol would be better for him than others, as well as the quantity and frequency of consumption that his body could best support.

You can see how a comprehensive approach that touches on almost all aspects of life creates the best opportunity for optimized longevity. There is no single supplement you can take, or activity you can engage in, that will give you a longer healthier life. It has to be cumulative and include every aspect of who you are.

The test results give us the information we needed to focus on the details, such as prioritizing one supplement over another, or knowing that strength training would have a greater impact than running. The information we gather when we choose to take control of our health enables us to make better decisions now and as we age.

Most of us want to age well. We want to remain healthy as we age so that we can enjoy our lives and our loved ones for longer. In many ways, John is a perfect example of this. Without a specific complaint or a goal in mind (other than "losing a little weight" and "lowering his cholesterol a bit"), we were able to collect information that gave John a clearer focus on what he could do to improve his health as well as his chances of living healthier for longer.

The result?

Once we assessed all of the test results and put a plan together for him, John ran with it. He had a newfound motivation to optimize his health. Since he wasn't starting from a huge deficit, he didn't expect to see huge results. However, the last time we talked, he happily reported a 30 pound weight loss!

John's energy levels returned and his mood was better. He felt like he had better control over all aspects of his life, not just his health. In fact, he said he felt like he was 20 years old again!

He had already made many of the changes and was excited for his future. John was even looking forward to his next lipid panel to see how his cholesterol responded to all of the modifications he had made.

Now that he had a deeper understanding of how his own body worked, he could make better decisions to support it. He also found it easier to invest in himself, because he knew that what he would be doing would have a greater impact than any generic solution offered.

In one of our follow-up appointments, John also noted that his digestive health felt much better. He hadn't really realized it, but he did tend to get bloated once in a while and perhaps constipated a few times a week. Since he has been on his regimen and changed his lifestyle dramatically, he noticed that as a "side effect" his gut symptoms disappeared. I told him that I always tell people that the gut is the "tattle tale" of the body. If you are having some digestive symptoms, it is worth looking deeply into what could be going on so that we can get to the root cause of those symptoms. Now that he was feeling better, losing weight, and optimizing his health, that tattle tale stopped complaining because it was happier than ever!

Even more importantly, perhaps, John learned what his most important risk factors were and how he could follow them. He planned to do annual brain imaging to make sure he stayed on top of anything that could impact his risk for Alzheimer's disease. By monitoring what he considered the most dangerous finding, he felt that if something started to change, he would be able to catch it sooner rather than later so that he could shift gears and change things if he needed to. He also understood that monitoring his other health parameters like his gut health, inflammatory markers, and toxin levels were going to be key to making sure that his brain remained pristine on those follow up MRIs.

Ultimately, the biggest impact I saw in John was that he was more engaged and more excited about his health. While he was always interested before, now he really "got it" and knew what he needed to do. Seeing how some minor changes made such a huge impact in his overall well-being really ignited his passion for life in general. It put him in a position where that excitement translated to an enthusiasm to help his family and friends also enjoy the same benefits he was seeing in himself. John now expressed interest in learning about things he might never have tried before, like yoga and infrared saunas. He wanted to keep learning, keep discovering, and keep optimizing. He asked me, at our last visit, what this passion was called. I told him it was called rescuing your health!

To be honest, I get super excited when my patients get excited. There are days when I want to drive around with a giant megaphone attached to my car to share all this good news. If only more people with "normal," "unremarkable," and/or "insignificant" test results could know the potential they have to optimize their health and feel anything but normal, unremarkable, and insignificant. I can only begin to imagine how many lives would change for the better.

Optimizing your health and focusing on longevity is accessible to everyone. In this story we followed John as he went from "okay" to "great!" That could be any of us. John's story represents the possibility we all have to create healthier todays resulting in better tomorrows.

CHAPTER 12

RESCUE YOUR BRAIN HEALTH

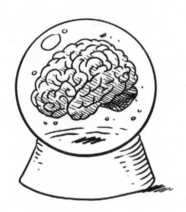

In some situations, we cannot take back the past. For example, if you had a traumatic brain injury and suffered some deficit as a result of that, we would never be able to promise you that it would be reversible. Similarly, if you have been diagnosed with Parkinson's, Alzheimer's, or multiple sclerosis, it would be wrong to propose that we could always entirely cure or reverse that diagnosis with the Precision Medicine approach. If someone tells you that's possible, it's more likely they are offering you hope and wishful thinking than truth. Don't get me wrong, though. If you've already been diagnosed, it's not hopeless.

We can still evaluate your risk factors and create a personalized protocol to help optimize them with the goal of improving longevity and quality of life. "Health" is not always about reversing a "diagnosis," because a diagnosis is just a group of signs and symptoms that certain people have that fit in a particular pattern. Different people get to that diagnosis by different paths; when we figure out what your path is, then we can try to make interventions.

When there is no diagnosis already, where we can intervene and offer hope is in assessing your risk for these (or related) conditions. Assessing risk means stratifying it, helping you understand all the variables, and making a plan for prolonged prevention.

When Brian came to me he was in his 30s and exhibited a few symptoms that had previously been diagnosed as migraines and IBS. He was told that his risk factors for these symptoms were the concussions he got from playing football when he was younger. He admits that a few times he "took a pretty big hit to the head." Again, his intuition said to dig a little deeper because something felt "off." What were his symptoms?

Upon our first meeting, here is what Brian reported:

- Fatigue
- Some weakness in some extremities
- Headaches
- Mild depression
- Brain fog
- Constipation

It seems like a diagnosis of "migraines" and "IBS" would make sense, based on this list. Sort of. The addition of "some weakness in some extremities" warranted a closer look. Brian also reported mild depression and was experiencing emotional distress because he was potentially going to lose his job, which required him to be physically healthy. Eventually, he had an MRI, and was diagnosed with multiple sclerosis.

Brian's symptoms pointed me to select tests that focused on his brain health and neurological risk. He also needed to stay within a specific budget. One of the benefits of using precision medicine is that you can tailor it to fit almost any budget, while still focusing on a specific area of concern.

Often, I feel like medicine uses a broad brush when trying to diagnose disease from an array of symptoms. More often than not, testing is done to "rule out" one thing or another, whereas precision medicine does the reverse. It assesses how different systems work, which then allows us to target interventions more specifically, thereby improving quality of life and well-being.

To accommodate Brian's budget, we focused on the tests that would be the most effective and give us the highest yield of information. Specifically, we investigated his:

- Mitochondrial function
- Toxin and mold levels
- Nutritional deficiencies
- Nutritional genetics
- Gut microbiome

Once we received his results, it became clear that there were external factors influencing his well-being, including potentially causing or exacerbating his symptoms. The biggest discovery was the level of toxins in his system. Brian's line of work had him exposed to numerous environmental toxins, which were most likely causing or contributing to his state of fatigue and headaches. Additionally, we discovered that he had mitochondrial dysfunction, which was not surprising given his previous diagnoses. However, we also found that his gut microbiome was tilted toward inflammation with evidence of intestinal permeability or leaky gut.

In short, Brian's body was struggling to keep up with the onslaught of toxins from his work, and it showed. The fact that he had taken several hits to the head when he was younger likely meant that the brain was a prime location for inflammation to settle in, because it was one of the more vulnerable parts of his body.

We concluded that it was possible that some of the toxic exposures he had experienced were contributing to the inflammatory state of his brain. When coupled with his history of concussion and traumatic brain injury, it seems plausible that he would be more susceptible to neuroinflammation. Unfortunately, there is no specific test that can test this exact theory, although there are tests that might suggest there is a degree of leakiness in the brain. We felt, however, that we had enough information to start putting together a protocol for him. It seems entirely plausible that these factors were all contributing to his health issues, and specifically his brain health. Before we finalized our protocol, we needed to know what else was affecting Brian.

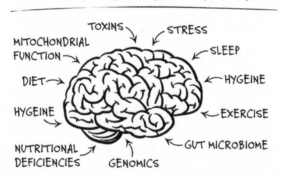

THINGS THAT CAN IMPACT BRAIN HEALTH

Upon reviewing his history, he reported high levels of stress, "adequate" sleep at around five hours a night, and an average diet that had room for improvement. When combined with the results from his toxicity screening, it all added up to the symptoms he was experiencing. His body was challenged to keep up with the toxin load, and his behaviors didn't help.

Given that Brian was a young, active individual, it seemed as though we had an opportunity to really make a big impact in his life with minimal interventions. The test results showed us where to focus our efforts in order to optimize his health and situation. I knew that with a few behavioral changes, Brian could experience a greater sense of well-being than he had in years.

To begin with, we put him on a regimen of probiotics, prebiotics, and serum-derived bovine immunoglobulin. This was to help him with his leaky gut, or intestinal permeability. The bigger issue was how we addressed his toxin load.

In order to help his body address the high levels of toxicity, I suggested a specific combination of supplements, some of which included: liposomal glutathione, milk thistle, vitamin c, omega 3s, and curcumin, among others. I also reviewed his vitamin levels, and specifically checked his Vitamin D and Vitamin B levels, making adjustments where necessary with the right supplements. This also helped support his mitochondrial health.

Since Brian reported higher than average stress levels, I suggested ashwagandha as well as breathing exercises. Specifically, I recommend the 4-7-8 breath, which can be found in the Appendix of this book. With these tools and interventions alone, Brian would have done well, but we took it a step further. After practicing the breathing technique for a while, we discussed the concepts of mindfulness and meditation. This was something he could add to his practice as he progressed, to further support his body and health.

We also had to address Brian's diet and sleep behaviors. In order to help his mitochondrial health as well as his sleep, we added melatonin to his regimen. Five hours of sleep is realistically too little for most people. There is a reason that the recommended amount of sleep is seven to eight hours per night. Consistently sleeping less than this will result in prolonged sleep deficit, which ultimately has a negative impact on health, including elevated stress and imbalances in the gut microbiome that favor an inflammatory state.

Finally, to alleviate his issues with constipation, I recommended triphala as well as ginger for bloating and to support his gut motility. The final suggestion was to continue exercising and to begin enjoying an infrared sauna on a regular basis.

This may seem like a lot, and for some people it may feel overwhelming to make so many changes at one time. Keep in mind that Brian was already diagnosed with multiple sclerosis, which meant that we had more than just a little bit of work to do in order to get control over the situation.

Again, this is why precision medicine is so powerful, because it's adaptive. Brian was capable of making all these changes, whereas someone else may not be. We always take sustainability into account when putting together a tailored plan for each patient. Some need to add pieces, bit by bit, and some need to do it all at once. Everyone's behavior profile is different, and it's included in the assessment of interventions. I always tell my patients that there is no rush. This is not a race. This is about your life, so we have all the time we need!

For Brian, he was ready and very eager to make the changes he needed to embrace in order to feel better. After only three months, he reported the following improvements to his health:

- Decreased anxiety
- Improved sleep
- Regular bowel movements
- Increased consumption of fruits and vegetables
- Elimination of brain fog
- Improved energy

Overall, Brian reported being much happier and feeling a lot better. He even shared that he noticed remarkable improvements in the first month alone. Brian had embraced the supplement and lifestyle changes and saw results. He felt optimistic that he would continue to improve, which became highly motivating. His plan was to work on other aspects of his health as he continued to feel better. Ultimately, he felt so much happier that he confided in me that he was planning to change professions to learn how to help people himself. I couldn't ask for a better result.

In the end, his original diagnoses were a place to start, not a place to end. Too often, I have seen patients who come to me with a diagnosis that feels like a death sentence. For neurological health, we know we can't reverse disease that has already progressed, but we can help prolong its onset or more severe symptoms. We do this by assessing personal risk using the tests I have mentioned above. For Brian, we hope that the changes he is making today will delay any potential progression of MS symptoms well into his future or even halt the disease process and allow him to have a better quality of life.

By taking the precision-based approach, we can dissect why someone is having certain issues or symptoms. When we put that together with imaging findings of the brain, we get a much clearer and more detailed picture of what can be done.

Knowing what's possible is the first step to rescuing your health. Applying it is the second.

Some people may find it scary to know their risk of developing Parkinson's, for example. I take the approach that if you know it now, you have a much better chance of changing behaviors that could delay its onset or severity. This could mean the difference allowing you to walk your daughter down the aisle on her wedding day, or to see your grandson get married.

By knowing your personal risk you can make decisions based on your own health profile, instead of only following protocols from the population-based risk assessments. Having a more precise and accurate viewpoint allows you to make decisions that can directly improve your quality of life for longer.

In Brian's case, we quickly saw a change in his quality of life. By identifying factors that could be driving inflammation in his brain, we were able to figure out strategies to address those factors. He not only saw this, but he felt its effects...in real time.

I will always remember what he told me the last time we met. He said "Doc, I want to thank you. You really changed my life. I know I have a long road ahead of me and I have a lot of work to do, but you really opened my eyes to realizing how much my environment and lifestyle choices impact my quality of life. I never really realized this until I started working at addressing these things."

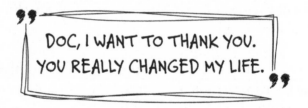

DOC, I WANT TO THANK YOU.
YOU REALLY CHANGED MY LIFE.

As a doctor, I could see it in his face as well. I could see that he didn't have bags under his eyes and that he was more alert and attentive during our follow-up visits. (Once in one of our earliest visits, he had actually almost dozed off sitting in the chair while talking to me!)

This was a new Brian. This was a Brian who not only realized what it means to rescue his health, but also one that appreciated it so much that he wanted to change careers so that he could teach what he learned to others. To me, this is what Precisionomics is really all about!

CHAPTER 13

Rescue Your Immune System (from Chronic Inflammation)

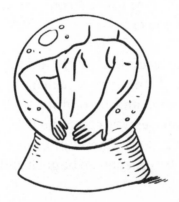

In today's world, we hear a lot about inflammation. Whether it's from the medical community, the fitness community, the self-help community, or the supplements/nutrition community, inflammation seems to be on the tip of everybody's tongues. So what is inflammation, really?

- Inflammation is the body's natural response to injury or infection.
- Inflammation is protective.
- Inflammation is typically localized to a specific area.

We need inflammation. Without it, we wouldn't be able to heal from wounds or infections. The inflammation I just described is *healthy* inflammation, and if we didn't have it, we would be much worse off.

Systemic chronic inflammation is different.

Systemic chronic inflammation is like turning the faucet on and never turning it off. You may need the hose to put out a fire, but if you leave it on, you may end up drowning instead.

When the body is in a state of systemic chronic inflammation, it can result in a wide variety of symptoms and diseases. More often than not, inflammation is considered "idiopathic." This simply means that we, as doctors, don't know its genesis or point of origin. We don't know *where* it comes from or *why* you have it, we just know that you do.

This means that systemic chronic inflammation is typically managed, not cured. This type of patient presents with a certain pattern of symptoms and laboratory findings that prompt a diagnosis and management plan. The interventions are largely aimed at reducing the inflammation in order to reduce the symptoms. These treatments can be great and even life-changing.

Just a few of the diseases associated with systemic chronic inflammation include:

- Rheumatoid Arthritis
- Lupus
- Fibromyalgia
- Inflammatory Bowel Disease (IBD)

Additionally, many of the symptoms experienced by people with systemic chronic inflammation include:

- Food intolerances
- Chronic pain
- Chronic gut issues
- Dermatologic issues

Over time, these symptoms can change. We often find that as the body builds a tolerance to a particular intervention or treatment, the symptoms begin to return. Managing systemic chronic inflammation is never a one-stop option. Unfortunately, by focusing on treating the symptoms, we rarely get to the underlying cause of the inflammation. This is frustrating for the physician, but even more so for the patient.

Most of the patients I have seen with this particular issue want to know *why* they have developed it, *what* they could have done differently to prevent it (or could do differently to manage it), and *how* they can reverse it, if possible.

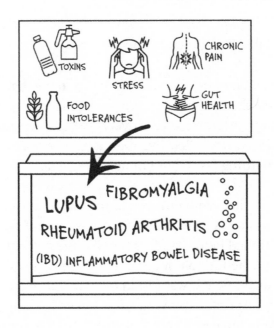

In order to help someone optimize their health, it's important to give them answers that provide actionable steps. In my opinion, the key to properly addressing systemic chronic inflammation is to do the detective work necessary to understand where it comes from so that you can know how to treat it.

When I first met Jennifer, she presented with the following list of symptoms and diagnoses:

- Chronic Fatigue
- Fibromyalgia
- Rheumatoid Arthritis
- Mixed Connective Tissue Disease (MCTD)
- Brain fog
- Whole body pains
- Constipation
- Joint aches and stiffness
- Low energy
- Irritable Bowel Syndrome

As a woman in her 60s, Jennifer expressed to me that she "simply didn't feel like she used to when she was younger." I have heard that phrase from numerous patients over the years, regardless of their age. They simply don't "feel like they used to," which translates to "I know something is off, but I'm not sure what."

After reviewing her symptoms and history, we focused on Jennifer's primary complaints: constipation and chronic gut symptoms. As I have mentioned before, I often say that the gut is the tattle tale of the body; when it's off, it could be a sign that something else is off in your body. We want to know what is going on in these major categories before moving forward and looking at anything else, especially since we know that 70-80% of the immune system is located in the gut.

The key to our approach is to look at factors that drive chronic inflammation. If we can address those—and optimize the gut microbiome in the process—then perhaps we can reduce the inflammation occurring in the gut to a point where we encourage the body to stop its systemic inflammatory response. For Jennifer, we started with these tests:

- Gut microbiome
- Food sensitivities
- Nutritional genetics
- Basic toxin screen

When we received the results, it was clear that Jennifer had gut dysbiosis and there was evidence of SIBO (Small Intestinal Bacterial Overgrowth). Dysbiosis is another way of saying "microbial imbalance." Knowing that this was the place to start before looking at anything else, we started her on a regimen of herbs. A 2014 study outlined how herbal therapies are just as effective as antibiotics for this specific condition.[55] In my experience, this has proven to be true.

Since SIBO can be a contributory factor in the development of intestinal permeability (leaky gut), we addressed this condition by first treating her for SIBO. After we successfully completed that treatment, we created a scheduled and prioritized approach to help support the rest of her intestinal imbalances and to bring the microbiome to a stable point after the herbal therapies we gave her. This included a spore-based probiotic, a prebiotic, L-glutamine, digestive enzymes, digestive bitters, and more.

We also focused on making some specific recommendations on how she could optimize her diet based on her microbiome and nutritional genetics results. This was particularly helpful for her, because she started to notice an immediate improvement within one month of changing her eating style.

---

55   Chedid V, Dhalla S, Clarke JO, et al. Herbal therapy is equivalent to rifaximin for the treatment of small intestinal bacterial overgrowth. Glob Adv Health Med. 2014;3(3):16-24, https://www.ncbi.nlm.nih.gov/pmc/articles/PMC4030608/

When a patient presents with idiopathic systemic inflammation, the cause can be related to any host of issues. For some it may be mold exposure. For others it could be gluten or a different food sensitivity. In general, however, I have found that it is usually a combination of factors that are driving the inflammation. It's never so simple that only one thing would be going on (remember the snow globe analogy?).

Therefore, the best place to start looking is by focusing on the symptoms—especially the chronic symptoms—that are causing the most distress to the patient. It's important to do this first because it can be harder to work on the long-term issues when someone is uncomfortable or not feeling well. By intervening on the most distressing symptoms, we create space for the patient to be more involved and invested in their well-being.

Once Jennifer identified her gut symptoms as the most concerning, we had a place to start. By honing in on this area, we were able to identify a potential cause and implement a strategy that would have the greatest impact on improving her quality of life.

Happily, Jennifer reported remarkable improvement. In fact, she improved much more than I had honestly anticipated. In only 2-3 months' time, Jennifer told me that

- her joint aches and stiffness had resolved,
- she no longer had brain fog, and
- her energy levels had increased dramatically.

At that point, she was a firm believer in the microbiome and was very happy with her outcome. So much so that, a few months later when she experienced a bout of sickness prompted by gastroenteritis and some of her old symptoms returned, she asked to repeat the microbiome test in order to address this new imbalance. With new information, her regimen was adjusted, and she was back on track in no time.

This is very important to note: the microbiome is not static. It is dynamic. It changes in response to what you have going on. Even though it wants to be in a state of homeostasis, the microbiome is always shifting. Life happens. You might get sick, like Jennifer did, or experience an injury and require antibiotics, or eat the wrong food, or suffer some other life trauma or stress. We all do. That's part of being human and living on planet Earth. So if you want to really keep on top of things, it is important to periodically peek in on those microbes so that you can see what they are up to.

When life happens, it's most important to remember two things:

1. Perspective: You view it as an obstacle you can overcome, not a life-sentence; and
2. Action: You use all the tools available to you to get back on track.

Gut microbiome testing is one of those tools.

By testing regularly, and acting on the results of such testing, we have a greater chance of ensuring that any temporary changes remain just that—temporary—rather than becoming a chronic problem, as is the nature of systemic inflammation and autoimmunity.

Additionally, I like to remind people that everyone is on a different path, and on a different trajectory. Jennifer responded very nicely, and very quickly. Someone else may take a year to make that same progress. So, it is important to not get frustrated and to keep on persevering. Some of the greatest accomplishments my patients have made took the most patience and persistence to achieve!

Through taking a precision approach, Jennifer created an opportunity for herself to learn that the answers to the questions she was asking were found right inside her body. She just had to know where to look and what to listen to. Once she did that, and once we helped translate that language into terms she could understand, she knew how to rescue her health.

Jennifer figured out what triggered her symptoms and how she could manage them better. She also figured out what she could do when she had a flare up that didn't respond well enough to her initial interventions. She became the boss of her own body, and she was very happy about that.

This experience also taught me that when we deal with chronic inflammation and focus on the main things that can influence it, we might end up getting more than we bargained for. By addressing gut health and her digestion, Jennifer also found that her systemic symptoms, like arthritis and fatigue, improved.

Even though we didn't build an initial program specifically for "fatigue," by working on the gut and her lifestyle we were able to lift that fog from over her head as well. What a wonderful side effect!

In the end, Jennifer had a new lease on life, and I was so honored that I could help her to realize the impact Precisionomics could have on her health.

CHAPTER 14

RESCUE YOUR HORMONES

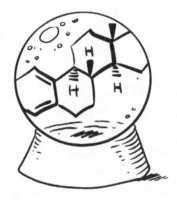

We've all been there. Work, life, more work, etc. It's a seemingly endless cycle that results in us feeling run down. But sometimes, that "run down" feeling is not the same as it usually is. Sometimes we have a sense that something is "off" even though we can't put our finger on it.

This is often the story I hear from patients who are eventually diagnosed with a hormone imbalance. Of course, there are also asymptomatic hormone imbalances that are caught with annual screening. Either way, hormone imbalance can eventually lead to feelings of low energy, anxiety, loss of libido, and general malaise.

Interestingly, most hormone imbalances can seem to "come out of nowhere." Someone who appears healthy, and who eats a healthy diet, may suddenly be diagnosed with hormone imbalance simply because something tipped the scales just enough for it to register. On the surface, many people with a hormone imbalance can appear to be doing well. It's only when something feels "off" that tests are conducted leading to a diagnosis. Prior to having concrete results, however, hormone imbalances can sometimes be attributed to other things, such as anxiety. Unfortunately, left unchecked, hormone imbalances can be rather disruptive to our lifestyles.

So, what causes a hormone imbalance?

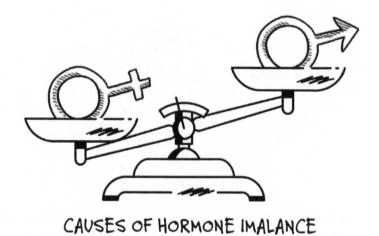

CAUSES OF HORMONE IMALANCE

In reality, there are many things that can contribute to hormone imbalance, such as gut microbiome, nutrition, and nutrient levels. For example, alterations in circulating estrogens can contribute to many different chronic conditions, including: obesity, metabolic syndrome, cancer, polycystic ovary syndrome, heart disease, and impaired brain function.

Additionally, the gut microbiome plays a key role in hormone balance—or imbalance.[56] In fact, gut health and hormone (endocrine) health are the same thing in my eyes. The gut

56   Baker JM, Al-Nakkash L, Herbst-Kralovetz MM. Estrogen-gut microbiome axis: Physiological and clinical implications. Maturitas. 2017 Sep;103:45-53, https://www.ncbi.nlm.nih.gov/pubmed/28778332

microbiome is an organ system that contributes to the regulation of our metabolism.[57] The metabolites (or products) that the bacteria in our gut make can act as factors that regulate our metabolism as well as a whole host of other functions in our body.

This was why I started by looking at her gut function when Sandra came to me feeling "off" and with a previous diagnosis of hyperthyroidism.

As a middle-aged woman, Sandra was busy with life. She was healthy, fit, exercised regularly, ate a lean diet, and kept a busy schedule with work. After she went on a major overseas trip for her job, she returned feeling more stressed than usual. Additionally, her heart rhythms became irregular. In general, she said she "simply didn't feel the same," even though nothing had really changed.

Her previous diagnoses included anxiety and menopause, until a blood test confirmed hyperthyroidism.

Knowing that she already had a diagnosed hormone imbalance, I conducted a wide array of testing that focused primarily on her gut microbiome, toxin, and micronutrient levels. Since she had been travelling internationally, she was already tested for parasites, as that could have been a cause of the sudden onset of symptoms. Her parasite tests were negative, so no intervention was needed in her case.

It's interesting to note, however, that an uncommon parasite—one that would not show up on the parasite test—could still impact the overall microbiome. As such, it's always good to test the microbiome when looking for a cause behind sudden symptoms. Additionally, if a parasite test is positive, that is the first thing treated before moving on to address (or test) any other systemic

---

57 Rastelli M, Cani PD, Knauf C. The Gut Microbiome Influences Host Endocrine Functions. Endocr Rev. 2019 Oct 1;40(5):1271-1284. doi: 10.1210/er.2018-00280, https://pubmed.ncbi.nlm.nih.gov/31081896/

issues, since removing the parasite from the equation may result in other systemic changes.

For Sandra, the tests I ordered included:

- Intestinal permeability
- Toxic exposure panel
- Food reactivities
- Nutritional genomics
- Gut microbiome

I knew Sandra was active and had a history of exercise and eating well, but we wanted to understand if her version of "eating well" actually matched what her body needed. What's considered healthy or "right" for one person, may not be right for another.

In our testing, we did not see flagrant evidence of leaky gut (intestinal permeability). We did, however, find significant reactivity to various chemicals, including phthalates and BPA. We also discovered that she was at risk for certain vitamin deficiencies and had an MTHFR mutation.[58] This gave us an idea that we had to focus on detoxification as well as supporting methylation. It also gave us a starting point to keep on digging.

There is well-established literature on the role that toxins in things like plastics, pesticides, synthetic fertilizers, electronic waste, and food additives can play in disrupting the gut microbiome.[59] In fact, we have a name for these chemicals. They are called endocrine disrupting chemicals (EDCs).

In humans, these chemicals are broken down by the microbes in the gut, and as a result we can see imbalances in blood sugar

---

58 MTHFR Gene, MedLine Plus, https://ghr.nlm.nih.gov/gene/MTHFR

59 Singh M, Mullin G. Diet and environmental chemicals and the gut microbiome. In: Vom Saal FCA, ed. Integrative environmental medicine. New York: Oxford University Press; 2017:115-40

management and hormones.[60] In fact, the microbiome regulates hormone systems and can influence many different aspects of hormone signaling. There is a two-way highway of communication between the hormone systems and the gut microbiome. Additionally, hormones can impact the richness and diversity of the gut microbiome.[61]

For Sandra, other findings included:

- A gene mutation that put her at high risk for hypertension and heart disease, if she consumed more than 1500mg of sodium daily
- Low levels of lactobacillus in her gut microbiome (a key type of microbe)
- Low level markers for inflammation and gut imbalance

All in all, we knew Sandra was experiencing symptoms that were negatively impacting her quality of life. We also knew that she had been diagnosed with hyperthyroidism, so we focused on how her gut microbiome, nutritional balance, environmental toxins, and lifestyle behaviors played a role in her situation.

By testing each of these categories and learning how her body was reacting to her behavioral choices, we were able to come up with an action plan that helped Sandra regain her feelings of health and well-being. Specifically, the goal was to restore balance in her various systems that support the rest of her body, thereby helping her hormonal imbalance. Just some of the personalized suggestions we shared with Sandra, based on her internal information, included:

---

60 Velmurugan G, Ramprasath T, Gilles M, Swaminathan K, Ramasamy S. Gut Microbiota, Endocrine-Disrupting Chemicals, and the Diabetes Epidemic. Trends Endocrinol Metab. 2017 Aug;28(8):612-625, https://pubmed.ncbi.nlm.nih.gov/28571659/

61 Williams CL, Garcia-Reyero N, Martyniuk CJ, Tubbs CW, Bisesi JH Jr. Regulation of endocrine systems by the microbiome: Perspectives from comparative animal models. Gen Comp Endocrinol. 2020 Jun 1, https://pubmed.ncbi.nlm.nih.gov/32061639/

Nutritional recommendations

- Intermittent fasting
- Detoxification using herbs such as: dandelion, cilantro, celery, burdock root, parsley, and red clover
- Sugar reduction
- Gluten avoidance
- Increase in fermented food consumption

Nutritional supplementation

- Selenium
- Curcumin
- Fish oil
- Magnesium
- Vitamin D with K2
- Vitamin C
- Probiotic
- Phytonutrients

Lifestyle changes

- Avoiding plastic bottles (many contain BPA)[62] (as it turns out, she was using these a lot during frequent travel)
- Green and Oolong teas
- Cultivating her meaningful relationships, and taking a break to enjoy life more
- Increasing sleep to 8 hours/night (instead of 5), consider using melatonin, if needed

---

62   What is BPA, and What are the Concerns About BPA?, Mayo Clinic, https://www.mayoclinic.org/healthy-lifestyle/nutrition-and-healthy-eating/expert-answers/bpa/faq-20058331

- Meditation 1-2 times daily (starting with simple breathwork practice)
- Increasing water consumption, ensuring filtered water
- Hiring a personal trainer for more focused exercise, emphasizing what her genetic advantages were
- Infrared sauna

This list may seem like a lot, but as we've already discussed, in precision medicine each list is personalized to the needs of the patient, and sustainability is taken into consideration alongside need and budget. In fact, we try to prioritize each list to make it easier for the patient to know where to start.

Additionally, the point isn't to do everything at one time. The point is to make it cumulative, by having it all organized as a roadmap that can be approached in a systematic, simple, and meaningful manner. You start with the easiest part (for you), and continue to build on it. There is no race. There is no rush. This is your *life* we are talking about, not just a *day* in your life, so we have plenty of time to help you rescue your health!

In Sandra's case, it provided her with the perfect roadmap to turn her life around. After about 6-8 months, she had done remarkably well. She reported feeling completely rejuvenated. While she still took a low dose medication for her hyperthyroidism, it was much better than it had been prior to her journey with precision medicine. She was happier, more focused, and back to her baseline.

In fact, in one of our later follow-up appointments, she said, "This protocol reversed my thyroid disease." She got a trainer, had more energy, and was having less body aches. She changed her diet and was reducing stress much more effectively. She realized that some of her toxic exposures could have come from a recent project in her house and she took action to mitigate them.

Ultimately, the way that she looked at life and her environment was different. She said to me, "It's like I had blurry vision this whole time and just needed the right pair of eyeglasses; now that I can see things better, I know what I need to do."

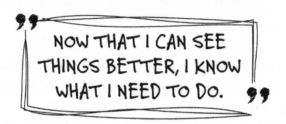

> NOW THAT I CAN SEE THINGS BETTER, I KNOW WHAT I NEED TO DO.

Knowing her health data was the catalyst Sandra needed to make informed, calculated decisions on her lifestyle, including diet and exercise. It gave her the upper hand in rescuing her health, and she plans to continue using this approach to further improve her quality of life and optimize her longevity and well-being.

As her doctor, I got to witness how this impact really changed her life. She was more calm and focused in our follow-up visits. Her anxiety had reduced. She was happier and full of energy. There was still work to do, but she now had the clarity and energy to get that work done. She was a classic example of my saying that "just like health and life can snowball out of control, it can also snowball into control."

CHAPTER 15

RESCUE YOUR REACTIVE RESPONSE
(TO ALLERGIES AND TOXINS)

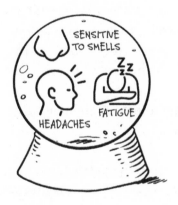

Why do certain people react to certain things, and other people do not? This question is at the core of precision medicine.

When someone has a reactive response to a stimulus, we often refer to it as "allergies." You may have hay fever, for example, which is known as a seasonal allergy. Or perhaps you are allergic to pet dander, or certain foods, like nuts. "Allergies" is our way of saying that the body has developed a reactive response to something you have ingested or is in your environment.

Allergies can be quite serious. There is a reason some individuals with severe reactive responses to a specific stimulus (nuts, or bees, for example) have to carry an epi-pen around with them at all times. That is not the type of reactive response we are addressing here.

The reactive response we want to focus on is the one that seems to have no specific origin. This is the individual who is prone to reacting to things like chemicals, foods, or smells. They have difficulty tolerating particular foods or food groups. They get headaches, experience fatigue, or feel depressed or anxious. They may even have sinus congestion or other allergic type symptoms. This person may also be prone to getting rashes, for unclear reasons.

Unfortunately, this patient is often dismissed or simply put on antihistamines or allergy shots. As a result, they may feel frustrated (because nothing seems to help), and they are often left with more questions than answers. Additionally, if this individual has food reactivities, they may be experiencing a very limited diet.

All of this directly affects their quality of life, which can feel confined and restricted.

While we look for underlying triggers, it's important to consider that a reactive response like this may be coming from immune dysfunction. Therefore, since the gut is at the center of the immune system, dysfunction in the gut could be largely contributory. Either way, the bottom line is that something is revving up the immune system, so much so that almost anything seems to cause a reaction.

This was exactly what Mark reported when we first sat down together. Over the years, his symptoms had increased until he finally reached a breaking point and wanted different answers. By the time we met, his symptom list included:

- Inability to eat a lot of foods
- Intolerance of meats
- Bloating

- Constipation
- High stress
- Anxiety
- Poor sleep
- Mood swings
- Frustration

Of course Mark was frustrated. Who wouldn't be? His life was being ruled by his inabilities, not by his abilities. When he came to me, he had been diagnosed with two conditions: IBS and GERD (gastroesophageal reflux disease). However, these seemed to me to be more of a side note compared to what was really going on. So we dug a little deeper.

When combining his diagnoses with his long list of symptoms, the only place to start was to do a full panel of tests, specifically looking at areas related to his immune system. Knowing that he was highly reactive, we were looking for the things that can drive a revved up immune response. Specifically, we looked at:

- Immune reactivities
- Food sensitivities
- Nutritional genetics
- Gut microbiome
- Inflammatory levels
- Nutrient levels
- Mold toxins
- Heavy metals

The result of all this testing pointed to dysregulated immune function. Until I started working with Mark, I had not seen someone undergo a food sensitivity test of 180 different foods and be reactive to 95% of the foods on the list—like I saw with him. I knew something else must be going on.

It seemed that Mark was what we call a "polyreactor." When someone is a polyreactor, it means that they have developed polyreactive antibodies, which could, in fact, be false positives. This kind of profile represents a larger picture of dysregulated immune functioning, which basically means that the immune system is reacting to everything, because something else is driving this reactivity. Therefore, the results that are showing positive reactions may not really be true. Sometimes this can be related to stress, microbiome dysfunction, intestinal permeability, or immune cell dysfunction.

Here are some of the major causes of polyreactive antibodies:

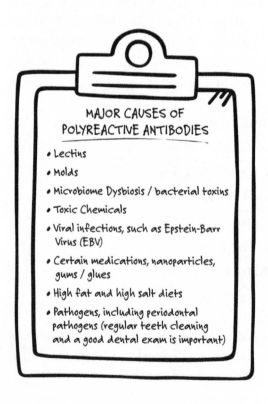

MAJOR CAUSES OF
POLYREACTIVE ANTIBODIES

• Lectins

• Molds

• Microbiome Dysbiosis / bacterial toxins

• Toxic Chemicals

• Viral infections, such as Epstein-Barr Virus (EBV)

• Certain medications, nanoparticles, gums / glues

• High fat and high salt diets

• Pathogens, including periodontal pathogens (regular teeth cleaning and a good dental exam is important)

For Mark, he had strong reactivities to ten chemicals and was essentially reactive to almost every food, hence the decision to look into these issues with more detail. The next step was to conduct more specific toxin testing as well as microbiome and pathogen assessments. In precision medicine, when we take a tailored approach, we can layer on the tests based on previous findings, or we can do many all at once, as in the case of John in an earlier chapter.

Interestingly, with the more specific tests, Mark was found to have some key deficiencies, and both his inflammatory markers and his homocysteine levels were quite high. Additionally, his environmental toxin exposure was elevated, which could have been due to his line of work.

Most importantly, however, Mark's tests demonstrated very high levels of six different mold toxins. Upon learning this, I immediately suggested he get an environmental specialist to evaluate the places where he spends the most time. This environmental specialist pursued the mold problem by conducting thorough inspections, and a major mold problem was, in fact, uncovered.

Mark was shocked that this problem had occurred without him knowing it. I reminded him that the most vital and urgent step to detoxing from mold is to get rid of the source or remediate the issue as soon as possible. No formal protocol is going to be worth anything if you are still continuously exposed to the problem. It was remediated immediately.

Knowing that Mark had high markers for many molds, toxins, and chemicals, as well as hyper-reactivity to a lot of foods, it seemed his dysregulated immune function could be attributed to underlying dysbiosis, toxicities, and a lot of stress. It was, in my estimation, a cyclical situation that continually reinforced itself, making his reactivity worse year over year.

In order to stop that snowball from continuing to go downhill and get bigger—and help Mark return to a healthier and less-reactive state—we focused on a protocol of interventions for both diet and lifestyle. Though it was both complex and comprehensive, everything was outlined in specific stages so that it was manageable. I also made sure to check in with him regularly to make sure he stayed on track.

For example, Mark was given multiple different diet directives to incorporate into his life over an extended period of time. This was supported with several different supplements to be introduced in stages to help with his process of detoxification and rebalancing his immune system. Examples of some of the things we used included: Calcium d-glucarate, digestive enzymes, digestive bitters, ginger, ashwagandha, liposomal glutathione, milk thistle, B vitamins, serum derived bovine immunoglobulin, and liposomal colostrum, among a few others.

Each of these choices were selected for a specific purpose, such as supporting digestion, balancing stress, supporting mitochondrial health, and detoxification. The focus was on ensuring we didn't overwhelm his system, which was already taxed and hyper-reactive. We had to introduce things slowly and give Mark time to adjust, because he was building health while simultaneously removing toxins.

A few of the simpler dietary and lifestyle changes that Mark employed included:

- Increasing water intake daily
- Ensuring proper fiber consumption (Mark aimed for 30-35gm/day)
- Engaging in regular breathwork and yoga or meditation daily
- Stretching calf muscles and increasing the duration of warm-up and cool-down periods before/after to working out (his genes suggested an increased risk of Achilles tendon injury)

- Avoiding high oxalate foods (peanuts, spinach, wheat bran, rhubarb)
- Eating calcium rich foods
- Drinking two to three cups of Oolong or green tea daily
- Avoiding processed foods and reducing sugar intake
- Journaling daily
- Using an infrared sauna regularly
- Performing one random act of kindness weekly

Even though he seemed to be starting from a more difficult place, Mark was starting, which is what mattered. Over the course of time, he found himself feeling more energetic. He began incorporating more ways to reduce stress and modifying his diet, which helped to manage his gastrointestinal symptoms and weight.

Mark loved how much better the infrared sauna made him feel, so much so that he bought one for his home. He was optimistic about the future and reported that he was looking forward to staying "one step ahead" in order to optimize his health for the long-term.

His quality of life was improving and, more importantly, he had an explanation for why he was feeling the way he was feeling. This is important to note because it went both ways. Not only did Mark have an explanation for why he had been feeling poorly, but he also had direct evidence of what was helping him feel better.

Mark knew that there was still more work to be done, but he was so glad to have gotten the opportunity to figure out the root cause of many of his problems. And, as a side note, his constipation also improved. He, too, experienced the simple truth that the gut is the tattle tale of the body. I knew that when his digestion improved, he was turning the corner and was going to be alright.

Over the course of his care, we reduced Mark's supplement use and got him on a solid regimen to help keep him balanced. Our plan was to monitor his toxin levels and to continue optimizing detoxification.

I would say that the biggest change that happened for Mark was realizing that our environment can play a large role in our health and wellness. He re-examined the type of furniture, clothing, and other items he purchased on a regular basis and started using trusted resources to help him figure out what personal care items were healthiest.[63] Finally, he started wearing a mask when he was on a job site where he may be exposed to certain chemicals and toxins.

Awareness is half the battle. If we are not aware about what is in our environment and how it is affecting our body, then we lose the chance to make an intervention. And that intervention may be something that needs to be done in order to improve your quality of life and overall well-being. I was happy to see that Mark was able to understand and appreciate this and even happier to see how his health improved once problem areas were addressed.

---

63 See Appendix for Dr. Marvin Singh's preferred list.

CHAPTER 16

RESCUE YOUR METABOLISM AND CARDIOVASCULAR FUNCTION

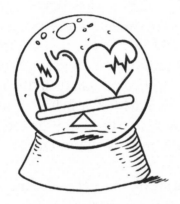

Metabolic imbalance is one of the more common complaints I see in my office. An individual with metabolic imbalance commonly presents with a cluster of symptoms that point to 1) an inability to lose weight, and 2) an increased risk of cardiovascular disease, diabetes, and metabolic syndrome.[64] There is often substantial overlap between this patient and other patient types, as many of the themes may appear to be common.

This is someone who is overweight, has a slow metabolism, possibly a fatty liver, and potentially has pre-diabetes or diabetes. It could also include someone who has simply tried and tried to lose weight, but cannot. Many times there are other issues like hair loss, hormone imbalance, sensitivities to chemicals or foods, and

---

64 Metabolic Syndrome, Mayo Clinic, https://www.mayoclinic.org/diseases-conditions/metabolic-syndrome/symptoms-causes/syc-20351916#:~:text=Metabolic%20syndrome%20is%20a%20cluster,abnormal%20cholesterol%20or%20triglyceride%20levels.

gastrointestinal upset. The reason for all this may be a common problem such as dysbiosis, or imbalance of the gut microbiome.

In this individual, numerous factors may be holding someone back from making progress, and there may be things you may not even think of to consider or that can't be tested, yet. For many with this profile type, life can be frustrating and every visit to the doctor can leave them feeling disheartened and even dejected.

Since there is no singular test that addresses every aspect of this list of symptoms, it is important to understand what is going on both medically and personally. For someone experiencing this array of concerns, the best way to find out what's going on is to gather data that is both scientific and contextual. In other words, the genetic testing will help point us in the right direction, but knowing what habits and lifestyle behaviors are at play is equally important, if not more so. This is why the extended conversation we have at the initial visit is so important.

For example, if you are overweight and cannot lose weight despite being on a strict low-calorie or fasting diet, it could be things like poor sleep hygiene and stress that are holding you back. Identifying these variables helps us find the best intervention. In short, all factors need to be considered and included when addressing metabolic imbalance.

When Sarah came to me complaining of stress and anxiety, we started by listing all of her symptoms, one-by-one:

- Hair loss
- Poor skin / Eczema
- Reactivities to chemicals
- Overweight
- General unhappiness

Previously, she had been diagnosed with IBS, a fatty liver, and obesity. While these may have been accurate statements or assessments, they weren't providing any answers or solutions. What Sarah needed was a comprehensive approach to health that was based on her own personal data. Going through another fad diet was not going to help her lose weight and keep it off for good. Understanding how her body functions—and what she could do to support it—would.

Our approach focused on clarifying what could be going on. We did tests for intestinal permeability (leaky gut), food reactivities, and inflammatory levels. We also checked her telomere length to gauge how much of a burden her DNA may be experiencing. We looked at her gut microbiome, checked her micronutrient levels, conducted several tests to evaluate for certain toxicities, and completed a nutritional genomics test.

After spending about half a day synthesizing all of the results and combining it with the information I gathered during our initial meeting, it seemed clear that Sarah had developed a pattern of gut permeability, inflammation, autoimmunity, dysbiosis, and toxicity. In order to help her reclaim and rescue her health, we focused our attention on these areas in a targeted manner based on the data we received from the various tests.

There were key components to the interventions we suggested that included both medicinal and lifestyle changes. For example, knowing Sarah's desire to make decisions that were sustainable, most interventions had to have a tangible approach. We suggested using "scheduling" as a major tool Sarah could employ to generate positive results. This meant:

- scheduling her exercise
- scheduling her meals (planning and preparing her weekly meals ahead of time)
- scheduling her social activities with friends

- scheduling date nights with her husband
- scheduling "me" time for her stress-reducing practices
- scheduling eating out 1-2 times a month (instead of weekly as she had been doing), to name a few

By focusing her efforts into using only one tangible tool in her approach, Sarah could plan for the changes she needed (and wanted) to make in a thoughtful way. We then used the information from her nutritional genomics test, microbiome test, and food sensitivities test to tailor a specific eating style for her. Again, we focused on a phased and tangible approach to help Sarah create meaningful and sustainable changes.

A few of the dietary interventions we incorporated into Sarah's health protocol included:

- Incorporating a targeted diet (such as Ketogenic) for a few months as a therapeutic tool
- Increasing monounsaturated fats (based on her nutritional genetics, this would help her with weight loss)
- Integrating detox-supportive foods, such as: carrots, parsnips, celery, cilantro, parsley, and dandelion
- Limiting high starch (her nutritional genetics suggested an decreased ability to digest and metabolize starch)
- Incorporating low salt diet (her nutritional genetics suggested an increased risk of hypertension and heart disease)

A few of the supplements we used to support Sarah's health improvement and optimization included:

- Fish oil
- Milk thistle
- Liposomal glutathione

- Vitamins C, D, K2
- Calcium supplementation

In order to support her improving health, Sarah also needed to make a few lifestyle changes. Our suggestions included:

- Avoiding excessive caffeine use
- Using an exercise tracking device
- Focusing on endurance activities (her genetic profile showed she was programmed to excel in endurance activities, such as fast-paced long walks)
- Using a hyperbaric oxygen chamber and infrared sauna, regularly
- Focusing on getting 7-8 hours of sleep/night
- Incorporating regular breathwork and mindfulness practice
- Planning travel to visit friends and family
- Using daily mantras
- Addressing stressors from early in her life and performing a forgiveness ceremony which I guided her on, in order to acknowledge her past while bringing closure to self-defeating feelings and emotions that continued to plague her in the present

Going forward, we identified additional tests that could be done to further refine our approach, making it even more specific to her needs. Good health is an ongoing practice, so it's important to have a means of assessing progress in order to redirect when needed. This can also be used to create motivation, as we have seen with all of our patients.

We had to redirect our interventions a couple of times with Sarah, because there were a few unexpected hurdles that came up, which is part of life. The key is to reassess, redirect, and keep going. We adjusted our approach, but overall we stuck to the general plan.

One hurdle Sarah experienced was the development of a rash which created anxiety around the idea that "it was happening again." This prompted her to take a step back in her progress. However, after we chatted about the rash and addressed the various possible causes, we realized that it wasn't a reaction to her regimen, but rather was a reaction to a new brand of makeup. We used this as an learning opportunity to reinforce the healthier habits she was creating and discussed the importance of sourcing good quality, toxin-free products. Once she stopped using the new makeup, things calmed down and she was back to baseline.

Over the course of a year, Sarah lost weight and both her skin and hair had improved. She stopped having reactions and her hair stopped falling out. She became motivated to work with a trainer and started prepping her foods several days in advance so that she could maximize her vegetable intake as she transitioned to more of a Mediterranean style of eating, with some modifications based on her internal data.

Sarah's sense of well-being was much better and she described herself as happier. She started hanging out with her friends again because she had more confidence in herself and no longer felt scared about being judged. Additionally, she no longer experienced bad dreams and was sleeping more comfortably at night. Her overall stress and anxiety decreased. Because of this, Sarah had the confidence and emotional space to address some stressors from her past and practice self-compassion.

Sarah was so happy with her initial results that she was crying happy tears in our follow-up sessions, amazed at how much her life had transformed. In truth, she became—in her own words—a "new woman." Her husband, family, and friends barely recognized her, and she was now living her best and healthiest life. In those follow-up sessions, we discussed how she had not become a new person—rather , she had become the woman she always was, no longer burdened by the symptoms of metabolic imbalance.

Sarah saw first-hand how, if you give your body the ingredients it needs to get the job done—the job that it wants to do—it will do the best that it can to protect you and keep you healthy in your environment. As a result, she was able to focus on her future, her career, and having children. She had avoided the topic of having kids before, because she worried she wasn't ready or healthy enough; but now she was excited and ready for what the future had in store for her and her family.

This is one of my favorite stories to share. It truly shows how important Precisionomics is when you are taking care of someone. Tests are important to guide us but they can't always paint the entire picture. Part of making sure that a precision-based approach is executed most effectively is in understanding the person in front of you.

Many of our obstacles to health and wellness are things we may not really appreciate until we invest in ourselves and take the time to dig deeper and investigate. As a physician, our success is dependent on giving the proper recommendations to someone in a way that they are best able to handle them. How many times has a doctor told you to "exercise and eat better" in order to balance your metabolism? What does that even mean, anyway? There are so many questions that need to be answered before you can truly help someone exercise, eat better, and balance their metabolism. Sarah learned this very well and is now a true believer in the power of rescuing your health!

CHAPTER 17

Rescue Your Gut

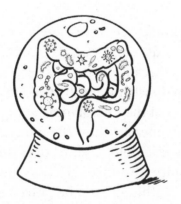

Gut dysbiosis is a more scientific way of saying "gut imbalance." More accurately, it means "gut microbiome imbalance." When the gut microbiome is imbalanced, a whole host of problems and symptoms can occur, as we have seen. In case you haven't noticed the pattern yet, the gut plays a role in practically every patient we have discussed. Even brain health can have its roots in the gut.

If you want to understand why you're having digestive symptoms, one of the first places to look is the gut microbiome.

The patient with an imbalanced gut microbiome could be someone who took a lot of antibiotics in their life, or it could be someone with chronic exposure to toxins and stress, or with poor sleep. In truth, it's probably all of the above in one way or another, and more.

Some of the key symptoms experienced by this individual include:

- Bloating
- Abdominal pain, problems digesting
- Inflammation
- Irregular bowel movements
- Food intolerances / Limited diet
- Fatigue
- Brain fog

We have great technologies now where we can sequence the gut microbiome and understand various aspects of its functionality. More importantly, because these tests are relatively quick and affordable, we can do what we really need to do and use them to assess the progress of the microbiome along the way. That is to say, we can literally measure how the interventions are working by seeing how the microbiome shifts over time. We can actually see the shifts resulting from a variety of lifestyle, dietary, and supplement factors. This, in turn, helps us stay one step ahead in rescuing our health. This is the point of Precisionomics.

Howard came to me experiencing many of the symptoms I described above, plus a few more. He was struggling with gaining weight and building muscle, as well as very high levels of stress and anxiety. Other than that, he also experienced unpredictable bowel movements, an intolerance for certain foods, and a lack of mental clarity (brain fog). Previously, he had been diagnosed with both Gastritis and IBS. When we first spoke, he expressed a desire to be "normal."

In order to assess his gut dysbiosis, we conducted a comprehensive evaluation that focused on the gut microbiome, food and chemical sensitivities, nutrient levels, and gut permeability, along with lactulose hydrogen breath testing for SIBO. We expected most of the results we received, which were: leaky gut, inflammation, toxicities, and SIBO.

We treated the SIBO using the herbal protocol previously described in Chapter 12 and added other gut-supportive measures, including natural therapies for gastritis and GERD, such as DGL (deglycyrrhizinated licorice), ginger, and slippery elm. We also incorporated digestive enzymes and bitters with Howard's meals in order to support digestion. To heal his leaky gut, we used probiotics, serum derived bovine immunoglobulin, liposomal colostrum, L-glutamine, and other supplements after the primary regimen was completed.

By focusing on supporting his gut microbiome in specific phases, we were able to address the majority of his initial complaints. However, there was more work to be done.

One of Howard's major contributing factors to his health was stress. Specifically, Howard was experiencing emotional stress—even duress—by holding on to difficult childhood memories. This was a huge factor that became more and more evident as we worked together and could not be overlooked. Even though we can help heal and support the gastrointestinal system with behavioral and dietary changes, if there is an underlying emotional factor, it too needs to be included in the treatment plan.

The gut-brain connection is definitely real. We know that stress can alter the gut microbiome and that the gut microbiome can impact how we feel, think, and experience pain. This bidirectional superhighway is active all day, every day, helping us sense stress and react to that stress. But when things become chronic (and/or related to suppressed emotions, as in this case), then the functions that are supposed to help us end up backfiring on us. Chronic stress can alter the motility of the digestive tract, or the way that the gut squeezes and moves its contents along. When the motility is chronically dysfunctional, then the symptoms that come along with it are often recurrent and ongoing as well.

Once Howard acknowledged the level to which his emotional stress contributed to his physical health, we focused on addressing it together. Releasing the stored-up fear, anxiety, and stress contributed substantially to his overall improvement. This release actually also allowed him to reconnect with family members he had not spent much time with and to heal old wounds.

In addition to this emotional work, in order to address any underlying causes of his gut imbalance—and prevent its return— we suggested Howard modify his lifestyle and diet. We initially started his dietary recommendations with a plan for intermittent fasting, low-histamine foods, and a ketogenic-style regimen avoiding FODMAPs (fermentable oligosaccharides, disaccharides, monosaccharides, and polyols)—types of carbohydrates strongly linked to digestive complaints since they are poorly absorbed.[65] He did very well on this regimen for quite some time. In fact, his microbiome data suggested that this would be the best eating style for him, so we went with it.

There was a time, about 6 months later, where we felt that the improvements Howard had made were great but had reached a plateau. We both felt like there was room for more improvement, so we checked in on the gut microbiome and did another test. It was only when we rechecked his gut microbiome that we realized a need to pivot away from the initial protocol.

While the ketogenic-style diet created a substantial improvement in his leaky gut and inflammation at that initial stage, it became clear that he needed more diversity in his gut microbiome, and he needed to increase the amount of plant-based foods he was eating. Howard was pretty nervous about making a change toward more of an anti-

---

65 Magge S, Lembo A. Low-FODMAP Diet for Treatment of Irritable Bowel Syndrome. Gastroenterol Hepatol (N Y). 2012;8(11):739-745, https://www.ncbi.nlm.nih.gov/pmc/articles/PMC3966170/

inflammatory/Mediterranean style of eating. I was, admittedly, a bit nervous as well, since he had been doing so well before. However, we both remembered one of my sayings—that the way we eat needs to be flexible and adaptable, and that as things inside our body shift and change, so do the things that our body needs to maintain optimal function. For Howard, we needed to increase detox-supportive foods and consider tighter fasting windows while moving to a plant-heavy Mediterranean style eating plan.

The ketogenic diet is a therapeutic diet. It has a role and a purpose. For Howard, that diet had served its purpose, and now we had to listen to what his gut microbiome was telling us. With the changes in place, Howard noted further physical improvements in both his energy levels and bowel movements in only a few weeks. He was shocked, and I was elated! We had encountered an obstacle, and we used Precisionomics to leap over that obstacle with great success!

In order to address Howard's desire to increase muscle mass and weight, we suggested he set realistic goals incorporating weight lifting and power-based activities, as well as resistance training. To further support his detoxification process, we recommended adding infrared sauna, increasing his water, and investigating some specific toxin sources we had noted by consulting with an integrative environmental medicine expert.

As he progressed, we also needed to circle back to Howard's other contributing factor to his gut imbalance: stress, or emotional stress to be exact. Our suggestion of optimizing family relationships, which we had already started working on, was a long-term goal that would take time. However, there were shorter, more immediate interventions he could incorporate, such as:

- Talking to his friends on a regular basis
- Finding a meditation practice that he enjoys, and meditate daily

- Improving sleep duration and quality, aiming for 7-8 hours per night
- Creating date nights with his spouse and incorporate family date night regularly
- Engaging in community service
- Continuing to take family trips
- Journaling regularly
- Replacing dysfunctional habits (such as chewing ice) with a breathwork practice or sipping herbal tea, such as lemon balm tea
- Considering EFT (emotional freedom therapy, aka tapping)
- Listening to binaural beats, especially when feeling a little stressed out

Howard was open to all of these suggestions, and other than a few flare-ups related to stress, traveling, or eating certain foods, he reported "life-changing differences" in his whole life and health. He started doing yoga and regular breathwork. His bowel movements became regular and much improved. He is happier, and his family life is significantly better. He even reports improved family relations over past issues.

Most importantly, Howard shared that he now knows *how* to handle flare ups. He understands *why* he has these symptoms and has the tools to address them immediately, making everything significantly less anxiety provoking. Howard is empowered and 100% rescuing his health.

Many of the supplements we put him on such as butyrate, a postbiotic and short chain fatty acid that helps reduce inflammation in the gut, were described as "game changing" measures. When we met recently, he said to me that "if I didn't have these protocols, I wouldn't know where I would be today. I don't know how I would have done this without your help and support. This is life-changing."

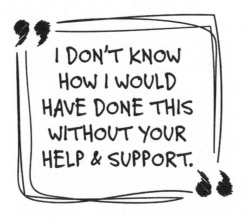

I DON'T KNOW HOW I WOULD HAVE DONE THIS WITHOUT YOUR HELP & SUPPORT.

This is so humbling for me because this is really what being a doctor is all about. This is why I went to medical school. Howard was more confident, less anxious, symptom free, and most of all, he was happy...really, truly, happy. He had a newfound excitement in life and was thankful that he was developing skills and insights that would help him and his wife with raising their wonderful children. This was really a case of Precisionomics at its finest!

CONCLUSION

The Journey Toward Greater Health

It brings me so much joy to know that someone has the tools and understanding to address their health, improve their quality of life, and optimize their longevity. We now have the science and technology to support this in ways we never have before. My patients usually come to me mired in frustration, fear, and feelings of despair. Inasmuch as my goal is to help them reclaim their physical vitality, I am most inspired by their willingness to show up and create change in their lives. They haven't given up hope, and now we have the tools to turn that hope into reality.

Precision medicine is a game changer in how we define health—or what it means to "be healthy." Instead of using statistics based on *everybody*, we now have the technology to go in and see what's true for you—*just you*. This means we can see how healthy you actually are, or what could use improvement, and make adjustments from that information.

It also lets us look at your risk factors for certain diseases such as breast cancer, heart disease, or Alzheimer's, and then make decisions to hopefully prevent—or at least prolong—their onset. Even more fascinating, we can also see where you might be prone to injury, which is definitely a game changer not only for professional athletes, but for anyone who regularly engages in sports or physical activity.

In short, precision medicine is our ticket to living healthier, for longer.

So, how do you start? That's a great question! First, search for and find a physician that you can identify with and that will be dedicated to helping you in the way that you need help. The doctor-patient relationship is a very important part of Precisionomics. Before your appointment, review the resources in the back of this book. Identify what areas of concern you have and what tests you might be interested in conducting. Then, when you chat with your doctor, talk to them about your health priorities and any issues (short-term and long-term) that you feel need to be followed, as well as what tests you'd like to have. Together, you can come up with an approach that will help get you started working toward your goals.

Some questions you can ask yourself include:

- If I were to fast-forward time and find that one year from now I was living my best and healthiest life, what would I have potentially done to get to that point?
- What is important to me?
- What is holding me back?
- What is my purpose in life and what keeps that internal fire burning?
- Why do I wake up every morning—what drives me?

Don't ever forget these things. These are the things that keep the wheel turning. We often forget about these things when we are stuck in the hustle and bustle of our daily routines. But, in fact, these are the things that make us who we are and give meaning to our lives. We can't forget that… ever!

Finally, as you get started on your health journey, it's important to remember that it's not all going to be beautiful music and roses the entire way. There may be some points in time where things are tough. As you've now read, most of my patients had periods where they had to readjust and redirect. Good health is not a "one-and-done" proposition.

Or, maybe everything will be smooth sailing for you and your journey will be one of steady progress. What's important to know is that every potential setback is a place to learn more about yourself; it's a place to figure out how to more effectively rescue your health. If you can learn about how your body is designed and learn how to maintain it and support it the majority of the time, you're doing well. Then, potential future setbacks may not be so bad after all; and if they are, you have the tools to figure out the problem, and the solution.

I tell everyone that each patient I meet is a puzzle… a puzzle where I don't know how many pieces there are and that I don't know how long it will take to complete. This can be challenging for the practitioner, but it's also a lot of fun because the end result is so worth it. And who doesn't like a good puzzle, right?

One thing that is very important to remember when putting the puzzle of your health together is that patience is a key factor to success. Patience and perseverance will get the job done. Remember, we aren't trying to run a race and see who can optimize their health the fastest. This isn't a competition. Often, when we do see rapid results, they're from a fad or extreme diet, which has little to do with "health" or wellness. Ultimately, wellness is about how you live, not about how you look!

This is your life we are talking about, so we have time. Take the time to get to know your body and how it works. Take the time to organize your questions, your symptoms, and your concerns. Take the time to write down your personal history, both physically and emotionally. Then find a physician who can (and will) take the time to get to know you, too. Then take the time, together, to make decisions on tests and interventions.

The investment you make in yourself is the one the reaps the most rewards. Once you do this, you will be well on your way to rescuing your health!

PART III:

PRACTICAL TOOLS AND RESOURCES

APPENDIX

In this Appendix, I have compiled some of the basic resources I use most often with my patients, as well as two forms you can use to get started in rescuing your health. My hope is that you will find these resources helpful. As always, if you are engaging in something new to help you rescue your health, please check with your doctor before beginning any new program.

Included in this Appendix:

It's important to me that you have usable resources and tools to help you on your journey. All of these resources and more are available to download on my website at www.RescueYourHealth.com.

HEALTH COACHING NOTES

In your own notebook, I recommend writing down these three prompts. Then, for each appointment you have with your doctor or other wellness professional, write your answers to each prompt. This will allow you to revisit key points along the way, without having to remember everything in your head.

Prompt #1
Things I want to remember from this session:

_____

_____

_____

Prompt #2
New things I can try:

_____

_____

_____

Prompt #3
Ways I can reinforce my sense of pleasure, purpose, and pride:

_____

_____

_____

MAP MY PROGRESS

Progress is a good way to reinforce your behavioral changes. When we see a tangible change, we know something is working. We then become more likely to continue with the changes we have made. Unfortunately, all too often, we forget where we started, so having a "map" to track our progress is really helpful. In your own notebook, I recommend using the following 10 prompts to record the changes you are making and how they are affecting your overall results, in real time. Then after a few months you can reflect, more easily, on where you were, where you are, and where you want to be.

1. **My Weight:**

   _____

2. **My Mood:**

   _____

3. **Average Sleep:**

   _____

4. **How I Am Reducing Toxins:**

   _____

5. **New Foods I Have Tried:**

   _____

6. **Foods I Have Eliminated:**

   _____

7. **How Much I Exercise:**

   _____

8. **How I Am Reducing Stress:**

   _____

9. **Fun Things I Have Done:**

   _____

10. **Friends I Have Connected With:**

   _____

The 4-7-8 Breath (The Gateway Breath)

This is my favorite relaxing breath. I learned it from Dr. Andrew Weil and use it often. I call it The Gateway Breath because once you feel how nicely this breath relaxes you, you will be interested in and curious about how you can keep that feeling going. Then you will be in a better place to learn more about different mindfulness practices.

Start by finding a quiet place and sit upright with your back straight and feet on the ground.

1. Close your mouth and quietly inhale through your nose for a count of 4.
2. Hold your breath for a count of 7 (in your belly, not your chest)
3. Exhale through your mouth with your lips pursed—making a "whoosh" sound—for a count of 8 (it's ok to be noisy here)
4. Repeat Steps 1-3 up to 7 more times, for a total of eight cycles.

THE 6 CATEGORIES OF LIFESTYLE MEDICINE: A PLACE TO START

Lifestyle Medicine is about incorporating all of the patient's life into the discussion and subsequent treatment plan. In order to rescue your health, a comprehensive approach that includes a lifestyle perspective is the best place to start. There are six categories in lifestyle medicine, as follows:

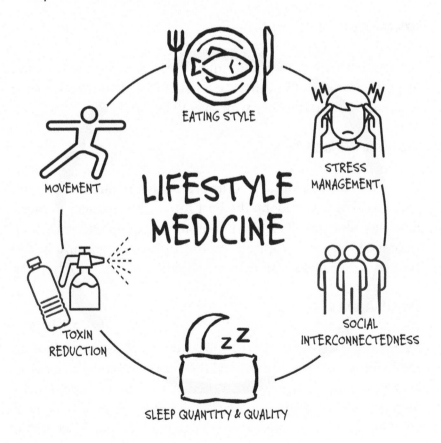

Eating Style

The types of food you personally need to eat in order to cultivate a diverse and resilient gut microbiome and optimize your genetic risk factors.

Movement

Exercise and/or movement. Whether you prefer to go for a run, go for a walk, or lift weights, the point is to get up and move. For every hour you sit, you should spend 10 minutes standing. Shoot for 150 minutes per week.

Toxin Reduction

You can evaluate your environment, see what you are exposed to, and systematically address any issues in order to reduce your toxic burden and improve your overall health.

Sleep (Quantity & Quality)

We want to target around 7 hours of sleep per night. There is data showing that this may be the best number to reduce all-cause mortality. Sleep quality is also important and we should be looking to reduce sleep interruptions, optimize the temperature in the room, and avoid electronic devices, lights, and other distractions.

Stress Management

Mitigating stress is one of the most important facets of lifestyle medicine. It is key to optimizing the gut microbiome and could influence genetic expression. Whether you prefer yoga, tai chi, qi gong, energy medicine, reiki, meditation, breathwork, or a combination of these and/or other modalities, the point is to spend time every day being grounded, being still, and appreciating the beauty that is your life force.

Social Interconnectedness

Humans are social beings. We need that social interconnectedness. The great thing is that we don't need 100 friends—we just need 1. We just need one person to talk to, confide in, bounce ideas off of. The microbiome responds to this as well, and those who live in areas where there is more social interaction and connection have more diverse gut microbiomes.

These six categories of lifestyle medicine are very important. They are the foundation of health. They are not to be underestimated. The beauty is that the treatments that come from focusing on these categories are essentially free (outside of food, which you have to eat anyway).

The human being wasn't built with a requirement to take dozens of medications. The human being was built with a simple instruction book. However, modernization and evolution of our species essentially changed how we operate, what we need, and what we develop in order to meet those needs. As a result, what we end up doing to our bodies also needs to change.

Therefore, in many cases, we may need to supplement or treat certain conditions. However, what remains true even to this very day in our advanced society is that the human body still responds quite wonderfully to these six principles of lifestyle medicine. When you give your body the things that it wants—the things that it needs—it will do the very best that it can under your circumstances and environment to be good, to be healthy, and to be in homeostasis. Why? Because that's what the body wants to do—that's what the body was meant to do.

Our default programming is to be good and healthy. By remembering the principles of lifestyle management in our everyday life, we can get back to that default programming. We can rescue our health!

The catch is that the body needs all of these things, not just one. You can sleep seven hours per night without interruption, but if you are eating chips and cookies all day long, you're not going to get anywhere. At the same time, if you eat plenty of vegetables and fruits and exercise regularly, you might find that you can now sleep better. Funny how that works right?

You see, the body needs all of these items in balance with one another in order to optimize health. However, this doesn't mean you have to work hard on each of these categories all the time. It's about balance and diversity. It's about incorporating some aspect of each of these six items on a regular basis to provide the best opportunity for your body. Then, the body will help you, because the body wants to get to the same place that you want to get to: health.

Dr. Marvin's Top Ten Foods

As you know by now, in order to optimize—and truly own—your health, the personalized approach is the way to go. Food is no different. However, there are certain characteristics that good foods contain, such as:

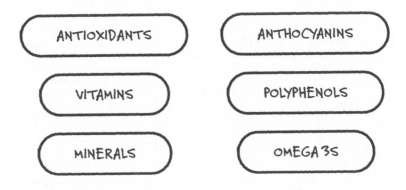

Of course, there are numerous other helpful compounds that you can consider as well, but this is a good place to start. Personally, I have a list of "favorite" foods that I recommend for their health benefits. To follow are my Top Ten Foods, including their health benefits and some suggestions for how to enjoy them.

Food	What are the health benefits?	How would you eat this?
Arugula	Source of calcium, potassium, folate, Vitamins A, C, and K. This more bitter or spicy tasting green may also help aid in digestion and can bring a nice flair to your dish.	• Mix in salad or add on top of almost any dish.
Asparagus	One of my favorite vegetables because it is low calorie and is a great source of fiber, folate, and Vitamins A, C, and K. Some benefits include: weight loss, improved digestion, and improved blood pressure.	• Chop it up in small pieces and throw it into a salad. • Grill it. • Sauté it. • Steam it. • Roast it with some olive oil and a little himalayan sea salt. • Add it into your stir fry. Just because it comes as a long-stalked vegetable doesn't mean you can't chop it up and use it in different ways.
Bok Choy	A member of the cruciferous vegetable family and a great source of vitamins and minerals. Provides a good source of Vitamins A, C, and K in addition to iron, calcium, manganese, and folate. It is also a source of sulforaphane which has anti-cancer benefits. Also contains brassinin which is an antioxidant. Also functions as an anti-inflammatory. Overall great for immune support.	• Sauté and eat it as a side dish or mixed in with other leafy greens. • Include it in a soup. • Grill it. • Steam it. • Include the leaves in salads.
Cilantro	This is a super-herb. Helps with detox-ification and blood sugar management. It is immune-boosting and filled with antioxidants which can benefit cardiac health and reduce inflammation.	• It makes a perfect garnish on many dishes. • It can be included in a smoothie or a cold pressed juice. • Liberally include this on a salad.
Ginger	One of my personal favorites. Good for nausea, bloating, motility, arthritis, reducing inflammation, reducing risk of heart disease, balancing blood sugar bal-ance, and it has antimicrobial properties	• Definitely can be included in cooking dishes as a spice. • May complement any dish as a side when it is pickled. • Can drink as a ginger shot.
Kimchi	One of my favorite fermented foods. Great source of probiotics. Low calorie. Boosts the immune system, reduces inflamma-tion, supports heart health, and might aid with weight loss. An acid in kimchi, HDMPPA*, may reduce inflammation. Get çthe gut boosting advantages and the nutrient advantages of this probiotic food and its spices, all in one package.	• Great side note to a dish. • Eat it as it is. • Mix it into a stir fry. • Mix it into a soup. • Makes a great complement to organic pastured, free-range, cage-free, antibiotic free, certified humane eggs.

Food	What are the health benefits?	How would you eat this?
Okinawan sweet potato	This purple-colored sweet potato is my favorite! High antioxidant levels make this particularly popular as a result of the anthocyanins that give the potato its purple color. Actually has more antioxidants than blueberries! Often mentioned as a food important in longevity. Good source of Vitamins A and C, Manganese, copper, fiber, B6, potassium, and iron. May have antibacterial and antifungal properties. Rich source of the hormone DHEA.	• Eat it like any other baked or mashed potato. • Cube it, roast it up, and eat it as a side dish with any meal.
Turmeric	This is a superfood with anti-inflammatory capability. Also an antioxidant. Can boost brain-derived neurotrophic factor (BDNF) and reduce risk of heart disease and potentially cancer.	• Use it as a spice on dishes. • Take a shot to get a turbo boost (often paired with ginger). • Many people don't know you can buy it in the store and it looks like an orange ginger. • You can steep your own tea with fresh turmeric.
Walnuts	One of my favorite nuts. Contains high levels of antioxidant capacity thanks to Vitamin E, melatonin, and polyphenols. Great source of omega-3s. Reduces inflammation with its Omega-3s, magnesium, and amino acid arginine. Promotes a healthy gut microbiome. May modify cancer risk and help control appetite and weight. Promotes brain health and reduces cardiovascular risk.	• Eat a handful raw. • Put on top of salad. • Add them as a condiment on top of organic, gluten-free, steel cut oatmeal. • Some like to make a nut butter out of them. • Some include them in smoothies.
Wild Blueberries	With 6 grams of fiber per cup, these are a delicious way to support your heart, brain, and gut health. High level of antioxidants. Low fodmap fruit. Some data suggests improvement in mood. Reduced risk of diabetes. Wild blueberries are believed to have higher antioxidant capabilities and have more anthocyanin. Good source of fiber, potassium, folate, vitamin C, B6.	• Eat them as they are. • Include them in smoothies. • At night, instead of ice cream, sit down with a bowl of blueberries with some cinnamon sprinkled on top to help with digestion, bloating, weight loss, and blood sugar control. • Pair them with a healthy nut like walnuts.

When trying to figure out what foods to include in your eating style, it can be really helpful to learn about what health benefits a food may have. I often do "food lessons" with my young kids. With 100% certainty I can tell you that, if I take a brand new food or a food that they don't care to eat and we sit down with the food, wash it together, and cut it together—and then quickly review what vitamins, minerals, and other great compounds are found in the food—I can't keep them away from the food if I try!

I remember when one of my children expressed that they didn't want to eat strawberries. We washed a bunch, smelled them, then sliced them in half. I told him about how there is a compound called fisetin in strawberries and this is an antioxidant that may help you live longer, promote good health, and help reduce allergies. On top of that we reviewed all the vitamins and minerals that are in strawberries. We discussed how food really can be medicine and that if we all eat these kinds of foods regularly, our body will respond by thanking us with good health. Then I concluded by saying you don't have to eat it if you don't want to, but at least we learned about the great health benefits of this berry. His response? "Of course I want to try it!" He ate one bite and immediately was sold!

This list of my top 10 foods are not all inclusive of the "best foods" one can eat. These are just some of my favorites. There are certainly many other foods I love as well as many other foods you can eat for your good health.

Nutrition is such a personal thing. However, there are some basic principles that apply to all human beings. There are some basic needs—vitamins, minerals, chemicals, and compounds—that we all benefit from. Therefore, I thought I would share some of my personal favorites that most people may be able to tolerate, outside of any particular allergies or specific digestive issues. I also wanted to offer a brief food lesson to demonstrate how food really is medicine if we think about its various components and attributes, and how we can use food and proper nutrition to reduce inflammation and optimize our health. Adding Precisionomics into the mix helps you go "next level" and truly rescue your health.

Now, just like I have favorite foods for health, there are also some "no-go" foods that it's important to know about, in my opinion.

A simple "Good" vs "Bad" food list isn't always helpful when we're talking about how you can optimize your health. Instead, it's important to look at—and understand—what's in the food and what it does to your body. Just like the strawberries in the previous section whose compounds help our bodies, there are certain compounds in food that actually stress our bodies. These are most often found in:

- Processed meats
- Packaged foods
- Trans-fats
- High mercury foods
- Sugary foods
- GMOs

While it may be a controversial topic, the literature does suggest that consumption of processed meats is associated with higher incidence of heart disease and diabetes.[66] While these studies might suggest a connection with nitrates, nitrites, and other chemicals, they also likely lack a comparison to organic meats, and further studies are likely necessary. In the meantime, it's a good idea to eat clean, organic meats whenever possible if you are going to include meat in your diet.

---

66 Micha R, Wallace SK, Mozaffarian D. Red and processed meat consumption and risk of incident coronary heart disease, stroke, and diabetes mellitus: a systematic review and meta-analysis. Circulation. 2010 Jun 1;121(21):2271-83, https://pubmed.ncbi.nlm.nih.gov/20479151/

On the other hand, it is more clear that trans-fats are not good for you and are associated with all-cause mortality (death from any cause), heart disease, and death from heart disease.[67] Foods that might contain trans-fats include: baked goods, shortening, fried foods, non-dairy coffee creamer, and margarine, to name a few.

Sugar-sweetened beverages are one of the most important things to eliminate from anyone's eating style, as they are a big source of added sugar and can be a large driving force in chronic inflammation. One 12-ounce can of Coca-Cola, for example, has 39 grams of sugar in it! This means that one soda, in and of itself, surpasses your total maximum recommended amount of sugar for the entire day, which is around 24-36 grams.[68] One recent study in the Mexican population suggested that consumption of soda was associated with adverse levels in a biomarker of inflammation called CRP (C-reactive protein) and cardiovascular risk.[69]

Of course, by now you know that nutrition needs to be personalized (and that we have the technology to do it). There are a lot of factors that need to be considered when figuring out an eating plan. The purpose of this book isn't to give you a diet but to open the discussion to the fact that your eating style might not be as straightforward as you think on the surface. After that, we can talk about how there are some certain principles to eating that are essentially important for all humans.

While it is important to figure out which foods are good—and not good—for you based on a variety of factors, we should all keep in mind that all of our bodies benefit from things like phytonutrients.

---

67 de Souza RJ, Mente A, Maroleanu A, Cozma AI, Ha V, Kishibe T, Uleryk E, Budylowski P, Schünemann H, Beyene J, Anand SS. Intake of saturated and trans unsaturated fatty acids and risk of all cause mortality, cardiovascular disease, and type 2 diabetes: systematic review and meta-analysis of observational studies. BMJ. 2015 Aug 11;351:h3978, https://pubmed.ncbi.nlm.nih.gov/26268692/

68 Johnson RK, Appel LJ, Brands M, et al. Dietary sugars intake and cardiovascular health: a scientific statement from the American Heart Association. Circulation. 2009;120:1011-20.

69 Tamez M, Monge A, López-Ridaura R, Fagherazzi G, Rinaldi S, Ortiz-Panozo E, Yunes E, Romieu I, Lajous M. Soda Intake Is Directly Associated with Serum C-Reactive Protein Concentration in Mexican Women. J Nutr. 2018 Jan 1;148(1):117-124, https://pubmed.ncbi.nlm.nih.gov/29378052/

Phytonutrients are plant nutrients with specific biological activities that support good health. Examples include polyphenols, terpenoids, resveratrol, flavonoids, isoflavonoids, carotenoids, limonoids, glucosinolates, phytoestrogens, phytosterols, and omega 3s. The compounds can act as antimicrobials, anti-oxidants, anti-inflammatories and may also play a role in diabetes, anti-aging, neuroprotection, and gut health—to name a few![70]

I think we all agree that things like Vitamin C and Vitamin D are also essential for human health. Vitamin C is an essential micronutrient for humans and is a potent antioxidant that plays a large role in modulating our immune system.[71] Vitamin D is widely viewed within the medical community as more than just a simple vitamin as it plays a large role in our immune and overall health. Specifically, it plays an important role in autoimmune disease, respiratory health, bone health, skin health, and gut health.[72]

So, while diet certainly is a personal topic, there are some common themes that hold true across the board. This discussion is meant to point out that there are some things that we know are universally bad for us and some things that we know are good for us. Understanding these concepts and combining this understanding with a personalized knowledge of your own inner biology… that's the special sauce to health and wellness!

A healthy diet considers all of these factors, as well as what you, personally, can tolerate. At the end of the day, a diet needs to be sustainable while also properly supporting the systems of your unique body. Remember, it all comes back to the systems. You wouldn't put diesel gas in an unleaded car, because the car's system isn't set up for that. Your body is the same. It has specific systems

---

70 Gupta C, Prakash D. Phytonutrients as therapeutic agents. J Complement Integr Med. 2014 Sep;11(3):151-69, https://pubmed.ncbi.nlm.nih.gov/25051278/

71 Carr AC, Maggini S. Vitamin C and Immune Function. Nutrients. 2017 Nov 3;9(11):1211. doi: 10.3390/nu9111211, https://pubmed.ncbi.nlm.nih.gov/29099763/

72 Bartley J. Vitamin D: emerging roles in infection and immunity. Expert Rev Anti Infect Ther. 2010 Dec;8(12):1359-69, https://pubmed.ncbi.nlm.nih.gov/21133662/

that are designed to work with specific components. It needs them to survive, and you need them to thrive.

When things feel complicated, I have found that it's always good to go back to basics. When thinking about your diet, after you have the information from your tests, a good question to ask yourself is this:

How far away from its natural state is this food?

Often, the further away something is from nature, the harder it is for our bodies to process it, which in turn causes added stress. It really is that simple.

Dr. Marvin's List of Key Herbs/Botanicals

This list is informational only and not meant to be prescriptive or comprehensive. There are many other herbs that can be considered in management; this list highlights some of the most popular that may help. Please adhere to any specific medical recommendations or advice and always do your own due diligence to ensure no drug-drug, herb-drug, or herb-herb interactions exist in your specific circumstances. And, as always, consult with your doctor before trying anything new. A great resource to learn more is the National Geographic Guide to Medicinal Herbs: The World's Most Effective Healing Plants.[73] The information contained here was adapted from that text.

BLOATING, IBS, SIBO

Constipation Predominant

Flaxseed herb - Used for: IBS-Constipation. 1-2 Tbsp. crushed flaxseed steeped in 2 cups water for 10 minutes; Strain, then drink through the day as mild stool softener.

Ginger - Used for: Nausea/vomiting, anti-inflammatory, gastroparesis, motility disorders, bloating with constipation predominance. 500-1000mg dried ginger twice to three times daily for gastroparesis before meals; 500mg twice to three times daily for nausea/vomiting. *[Caution: GERD (in some), pregnancy, high doses in conjunction with anticoagulants.]*

---

73 Johnson, R.L., Foster, S., Low Dog, T, and Kiefer, D. (2012). National Geographic Guide to Medicinal Herbs: The World's Most Effective Healing Plants. National Geographic.

Triphala - Used for: Constipation, bowel tonic, IBS, lower cholesterol and BP, antioxidant, anti-inflammatory. Take capsules, avoid powder. Follow the label for dosing, 1-2 times daily before eating. [Caution: loose stools, stomach upset.]

Diarrhea Predominant

Caraway seed oil - Used for: GERD, dyspepsia, antispasmodic, IBS-diarrhea predominant. 50-100mg or 0.2mL in enteric-coated capsule two to three times daily. 1-4 drops daily of essential oil.

Serum-derived bovine immunoglobulin (SBI) - Used for: Diarrhea, IBS, SIBO. Serum derived bovine immunoglobulin/ protein isolate, binds microbial components, toxic substances released by bacteria.

Peppermint - Used for: Indigestion, IBS with diarrhea, colds/ cough, muscle aches, tension headaches, bloating, improved bile flow, abdominal cramping. 50mg or 0.2mL in enteric coated capsule two to three times daily before meals; if anal burning, reduce and/or take with food. *[Caution: GERD, hiatal hernia.]*

Bloating/SIBO predominant

Herbal blend of peppermint leaf, quebracho extract, conker tree extract, horse chestnut - Used for: Bloating, abdominal discomfort, changing bowel habits. 2 capsules daily; take before foods that are bothersome and up to three times daily until relief attained, then consider 2 capsules daily once stable. *[Caution: Consider the length of treatment.]*

Berberine (compound in goldenseal) - Used for: Intestinal permeability, diarrhea, SIBO, antibacterial. 500mg two to three times daily.

Fennel - Used for: Colic, menstrual cramps, bloating, coughs/ cold/sinus congestion, abdominal cramps. *[Caution: use in pregnancy limited to what is found in food.]*

Uva ursi (bearberry) - Used for: Antibacterial. Tea, capsule (standardized extracts of 700-1000mg three times daily), tincture (1tsp three times daily). *[Caution: do not take longer than 2 weeks; not for children, pregnancy, breastfeeding, kidney failure; tannins can cause upset stomach, nausea, vomiting, constipation.]*

General

Chamomile - Used for: IBS, GERD, colic, relaxes gut smooth muscle, calms the mind, anti-ulcerogenic. 1-3 cups infusion per day, 3-10mL twice daily (1:5 tincture or glycerite), 500- 2000mg dried flower in capsules twice daily.

GERD

Aloe Vera - Juice or gel, Aloin free product. GERD, IBD, constipation, mucosal healing, anti-inflammatory. 100-150mL twice daily. *[Caution: GI upset, melanosis coli.]*

Caraway seed oil - GERD, dyspepsia, antispasmodic, IBS- diarrhea predominant. 50-100mg or 0.2mL in enteric-coated capsule two to three times daily. 1-4 drops daily of essential oil.

D-Limonene - GERD, ulcers, promote gut motility, stimulate gut peristalsis: 1000mg daily every other day for 10 doses over 20 days, then as needed. *[Caution: pregnancy.]*

Deglycyrrhizinated licorice (DGL) - GERD, sore throat, gastritis. 400-800mg taken before meals and bedtime. *[Caution: pregnancy.]*

Ginger - Nausea/vomiting, anti-inflammatory, gastroparesis, motility disorders, bloating with constipation predominance. 500-1000mg dried ginger twice to three times daily for gastroparesis before meals; 500mg twice to three times daily for nausea/vomiting. *[Caution: GERD (in some), pregnancy, high doses in conjunction with anticoagulants.]*

Mastic gum - Dyspepsia, peptic ulcer, H.pylori, antacid. 1-2gm per day.

Melatonin - Particularly for nocturnal GERD. Take 3mg two hours before bed.

Slippery elm - GERD, IBD cough, sore throat, itchy/inflamed skin. Lozenges for GERD, IBD, sore throat. Tea: steep 1 tsp powder in 1 cup water for 10 min; pour off liquid; discard powdered sediment in bottom of cup; drink 1 cup between or after meals. Tinctures should use low amounts of alcohol or mucopolysaccharides will be degraded. *[Caution: Can slow absorption of other medicines; should be taken 1 hr before or several hours after; not recommended with bile duct obstruction or gallstones.].*

Digestive Aids

Digestive bitters (including artichoke, dandelion root, gentian, hops, bitter orange peel) - Digestive aid, increases gastric acid and primes pancreas; bloating; gas; sluggish stools; fullness after eating; dyspepsia; IBS. Dandelion can be used for sluggish digestion and as liver protectant (1-3 gm of dandelion leaf/root taken in divided doses; tea or capsules). Artichoke leaf: promotes bile flow, anti-nausea: 320mg-640mg daily. *[Caution: allergy, GERD, increased stomach acid, gallbladder/ kidney problems, possible drug interactions.]*

STW5 (blend of 9 herbs) = Iberis, amara, angelica, chamomile, caraway, milk thistle, lemon balm, peppermint, celandine, licorice) - IBS, functional dyspepsia. 20 drops before or with meals for those aged 12 and up. *[Caution: allergy, liver disease, pregnancy, breastfeeding.]*

Liver Support

Dandelion - see "Digestive bitters"

Milk thistle - Liver disease. Standardized to 80% silymarin, optimal dose is not known; in Hep C and cirrhosis close is close to 700mg extract three times daily. Use as hepatoprotectant from drug induced damage. Beneficial dose 420-760mg daily in divided doses.

Anti-inflammatory/Immune

Boswellia - IBD, microscopic colitis, gut healing. Standardized to 65% boswellin or boswellic acid. 300-500mg three times daily (many use 350mg three times daily). *[Caution: nausea, diarrhea, rash.]*

Elder (elderberry) - Colds, flus. Syrup/lozenge. *[Caution: do not eat unripe berries or consume products made from other plant parts. Caution with autoimmune conditions.]*

Glutamine - *(not truly a botanical but mentioned here in brief)* for gut lining repair, IBD: 2-3gm per day

Marshmallow root - IBD, GERD. 6gm/day. Tea: steep 1 tbsp root in 2 cups near boiling water for 15-20 min; strain then drink 60 minutes after meals.

Turmeric - Anti-inflammatory, arthritis, IBD, FAP, prevention of cardiovascular disease and cancer. Standardized 95%

curcumin or curcuminoids. 300-600mg three times daily to 1500-3000mg daily in divided doses for IBD have been recommended. *[Caution: eating it is safe and high doses up to 12gm/dy are well tolerated although no*

Stress Reduction

Ashwagandha - Rejuvenating tonic, anti-inflammatory, anti-anxiety. 1-6gm per day of dried root in 2-3 divided doses; 2-4mL three times daily tincture. Tea. *[Caution: sedation, nausea, diarrhea, may stimulate thyroid activity; Caution in pregnancy; Caution with other sedating drugs.]*

Lavender - Insomnia, anxiety, gas, stomach upset, bad breath. Tea. Massage/oil. Aromatherapy. For mild digestive upset, add a few drops of lavender oil to a sugar cube and allow it to dissolve in the mouth. 5-10 drops to bath water.

Lemon Balm - Dyspepsia, gut calming agent, anxiety, colic. 900-1500mg daily; tea.

Milky oat seed - Restorative tonic, tensions/stress relief. Take 30-50 drops in a small amount of water 3-4 times daily between meals.

Passion Flower - Anxiety, insomnia. Infusion, tea. 1-2 350mg caps daily to twice daily. Tincture: 1-2mL daily to three times daily, often combined with hops or lemon balm. *[Caution: drowsy, dizzy, increased effects of other sedatives; Do not take in pregnancy; Can increase activity or interact with anticoagulants or blood thinning medications.]*

Raspberry leaf - Women's tonic (regular menstrual cycles and ease cramping), pregnancy tea, diarrhea. Tea, capsules (500mg to 600mg dried leaf 2-4 times daily), tincture 5mL twice daily.

Rhodiola - Stress, anxiety, depression, fatigue. Tea. Tincture 3-5mL twice daily. Extract: 100-576mg extract standardized to contain 3.6% rosavin and 1.6% salidroside. *[Caution: interaction with antidepressants and those with mental health conditions should consult a doctor first; Caution in pregnancy.]*

Memory

Bacopa monnieri - Cognition, memory, anti-anxiety. 5-10gm daily of powdered bacopa in capsules. Tea. 1-2 tsp of tincture daily or 2 tbsp syrup daily. Standardized extracts contain 20-55% bacosides; dosage is 150mg twice daily. *[Caution: dry mouth, nausea, fatigue, drowsiness with other sedatives, may interact with thyroid medications.]*

Gotu Kola - Memory/cognition, venous insufficiency, wound healing. Capsules: standardized extracts of 30mg total triterpenoids per capsule, taken in 1-2 capsules twice daily; total dried leaves, stems, flowers should be 0.5 to 6gm daily. Tincture: 2-4 tsp daily. *[Caution: liver disease or issues; Upset stomach, nausea; Avoid in pregnancy.]*

Sleep

Melatonin - Particularly for nocturnal GERD, take 3mg two hours before bed.

DR. MARVIN'S GUIDE TO SUPPLEMENT BRANDS

Supplements, like everything else we've talked about, need to be personalized. However, there are certain things that remain true, regardless of what supplement you need. Specifically, it's most important to understand how to choose a supplement brand once you know what you need and in what dose you need it. To that end, I've compiled a checklist of tips to help you navigate the supplement world with a little more information.

15 Tips on HOW to Choose a Supplement Brand

1. Do your research: https://drlowdog.com/resources/
2. Look for reputable brands, made in the USA
3. Look for 3rd party seals like United States Pharmacopeia, NSF International, Consumer Labs, Good Manufacturing Practices
4. Labels should not claim that a supplement treats or cures diseases
5. For a chart detailing the upper intake levels of vitamins and minerals, visit the NIH website (NIH.gov) or refer to Dr. Tieraona Low Dog's book Fortify Your Life
6. Check labels to see if capsules are made from veggie caps or from gelatin (animal source)
7. Softgels are almost exclusively from gelatin (from animal sources) and may not be suitable for vegetarians/vegans
8. Beware of sweeteners and/or flavorings in chewables (and lactic acid, which may be derived from dairy if you are a vegan or sensitive to dairy)

9. Taking large doses of Calcium (Ca) or Magnesium (Mg) can compete with absorption of other minerals, including each other; therefore, take Mg at bed to help with sleep and relaxation and take the MVI-mineral supplement at least 2 hours apart from Ca or Mg.

10. Best to take fat-soluble vitamins (A, D, E, K, fish oil) with food (in particular, with a meal containing fat—not a snack!)

11. Look at the labels to make sure you don't have specific allergies or sensitivities to any of the ingredients or fillers

12. Try to get Non-GMO, organic-based products, if available/possible

13. Key components of any supplement label should include: product name, manufacturer name, manufacturer claims, method of delivery, "supplement facts" or ingredients, serving information, units of measurement, percentage daily value (DV), other ingredients, suggested use, cautions and warnings, manufacturer's contact information, lot number, expiration date, quality seals

14. Supplements, herbs, and medical foods are not as tightly regulated as prescription drugs. Therefore, one must keep in mind that a practitioner cannot guarantee quality or purity of product at all times (which actually holds true for both prescription and non-prescription drugs); one must continually do their own research and ensure that products are safe for them, under their circumstances

15. Check for drug-drug, herb-drug, herb-herb interactions. One good site: https://www.umm.edu/health/medical/altmed but there are many others such as Consumer Labs, Sloan Kettering, etc

Note: This is simply a starter's guide and is not meant to be comprehensive or all encompassing. These are general recommendations for those seeking supplements or herbal remedies and is not meant to provide medical advice to any particular individual without expressed recommendations. And, as always, consult with your doctor before trying anything new.

What Tests Might Be Good for Me?

It can sometimes be tough to figure out where to start and what kinds of tests you might want to discuss getting done with your healthcare provider. This guide may help you streamline some of your initial choices based on your personal health priorities.

General Health and Wellness:
- Basic cardiometabolic tests
- Hormone panel
- Microbiome sequencing
- Nutritional genomics or whole exome sequencing
- Micronutrient testing
- Whole body imaging
- Body composition imaging

Brain Health:
- Leaky gut test
- Toxin testing
- Microbiome sequencing
- Basic inflammatory markers
- Mitochondrial health assessment

Autoimmunity:
- Basic inflammatory markers
- Whole exome sequencing
- Microbiome sequencing
- Leaky gut testing
- Food sensitivity testing
- Toxin testing

Hormones:
- Complete hormone panel
- Microbiome sequencing
- Basic inflammatory and autoimmune markers
- Micronutrient testing

Reactive Response:
- Leaky gut test
- Microbiome sequencing
- Food and chemical sensitivity panel
- Pathogen detection test
- Basic inflammatory markers

Metabolic imbalance:
- Basic lab testing: fasting blood sugar, insulin, TMAO, Hgb A1c, inflammatory markers
- AMRA body composition scan
- Microbiome sequencing
- Nutritional genomics or whole exome sequencing

Gut imbalance:
- Microbiome sequencing
- SIBO testing
- Toxin testing
- Stool calprotectin
- Fecal pancreatic elastase
- Food sensitivity testing
- Leaky gut test

What Supplements Am I Taking?

A simple chart like this might help you keep your supplements organized so that you know what you are taking, what it is for, and how much to take (and when).

Feel free to adapt this table and modify it for your personalized needs.

Supplement (By Category)	Dose (As Instructed by Healthcare Provider)	Time of day to take supplement (AM/midday/PM)
Gut Health		
Immune Health		
Mitochondrial Health		

Supplement (By Category)	Dose (As Instructed by Healthcare Provider)	Time of day to take supplement (AM/midday/PM)
Anti-inflammatory		
Detoxification		
Vitamins/General Health		
Symptom-Specific Supplements		

ACKNOWLEDGEMENTS

Writing this book has been so much fun! I'm really excited for everyone to read it and learn about how important it is to take a personalized approach to health and wellness. There have been so many people that have helped me along the way and brought me to the exciting place I'm in today. Without their help, this book wouldn't have been possible.

Thank you to my beautiful wife, Crystal, and my two awesome and amazing sons, Benjamin and Wellington. You have been my anchor, my rocks. Thank you for all the love, help, and support you have given me. Without your love and dedication, I wouldn't be the husband, father, and doctor that I am today. Thank you to my parents, Mohan and Harbans, who taught me the importance of kindness, compassion, and selflessly helping people from a very young age. Your wisdom, guidance, and love are unparalleled. To Kevin, Priya, Asha, and Kam, your love and support are what keeps me going! A heartfelt thanks to Allan, Sue, Stephanie, Danielle, Matt, Heather, Dave, Joshua, Mikaila, Owen, Brady, and all of my amazing family in Canada. The support you have all given me throughout the years truly warms my heart. I wouldn't be the man I am today without you! Thank you!

Dr. Gerard Mullin, my mentor and good friend, I owe you so much. Without your guidance and help, I may not have ever found integrative medicine (or myself). Dr. Andrew Weil, you have inspired me so much just as you have inspired thousands and thousands of others. Thank you for teaching me the value of integrative medicine and helping me understand that there is so much more to health than what we are taught in medical school.

Thank you also for writing the Foreword to this book. It means so much to me!

A huge heartfelt thanks to Martina Faulkner, James Tager, Mark Tager, Robert Hughes, Scott Sensenbrenner, Kiran Krishnan, Tom Bayne, Andrew Mills, Ahmed El-Sohemy, David Karow, Julia Craven, Matthew Formeller, Bob Jankowski, Chris Ross, and Shaista Malik. Without your help, support, mentorship, guidance, and collaboration, this book would not have been possible. I also have to thank Dr. Daniel Siegel and Dr. Shauna Shapiro; you two may not know it but you have made a profound impact on my life in teaching me about mindfulness.

As I am writing this, I realize that there are so many people to thank—more than I can fit on these pages. I have been blessed to have many fantastic friends, mentors, teachers, and colleagues. You have all been instrumental in making me who I am today and helping me write my first book. Thank you for believing in me!

Finally, and very importantly, I want to thank every single patient I have ever had the pleasure of meeting. You inspire and teach me something every single day. For that, I am forever indebted to you all!